Young People and Sexual Expl

Work with sexually exploited young people can be rewarding yet difficult. They can be hard to access, often presenting challenging behaviour. Sometimes it is painful to hear their life stories, whether these include abuse through the internet or exploitation experienced through having been trafficked into and within the country.

Jenny J. Pearce draws on young people's voices to explore the difficulties that arise for researchers and for practitioners when working with sexually exploited young people. While child protection interventions must guide social work, she argues that other agencies such as health, education, housing and training each have a role to play in supporting a sexually exploited young person.

Challenging the uncritical acceptance of the child as victim, the book suggests 'therapeutic outreach' as an approach to working with sexually exploited young people that can complement child protection procedures, support practitioners in the field and enhance the young person's sense of autonomy and responsibility during their transition to adulthood.

The book advocates the relationship between practitioners and the young people they aim to support to be one of the most important resources in practice.

Young People and Sexual Exploitation will be essential reading for anyone interested in preventing the sexual exploitation of children and young people. It will be particularly relevant for academics, students, practitioners and policy-makers in the fields of social policy and social work, child and family work, child protection or youth work.

Jenny. J. Pearce is Professor of Young People and Public Policy at the University of Bedfordshire; Director of the International Centre for the Study of Sexually Exploited and Trafficked Children and Young People; and co-founder/member of the National Working Group for Sexually Exploited Children and Young People

Young People and Sexual Exploitation

'It's not hidden, you just aren't looking'

Jenny J. Pearce

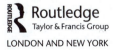 Routledge
Taylor & Francis Group

LONDON AND NEW YORK

First published 2009
by Routledge
2 Park Square, Milton Park, Abingdon, Oxon, OX14 4RN

Simultaneously published in the USA and Canada
by Routledge-Cavendish
270 Madison Avenue, New York, NY 10016

Routledge is an imprint of the Taylor & Francis Group, an informa business

© 2009 Jenny J. Pearce

Typeset in Sabon by Taylor & Francis Books
Printed and bound in Great Britain by TJ International Ltd, Padstow, Cornwall

British Library Cataloguing in Publication Data
A catalogue record for this book is available from the British Library

Library of Congress Cataloging-in-Publication Data
Pearce, Jenny J.
  Young people and sexual exploitation : "it's not hidden, you just aren't
looking" / Jenny J. Pearce.
    p.; cm.
  1. Child sexual abuse. 2. Child prostitution. I. Title.
[DNLM: 1. Child Abuse, Sexual—psychology. 2. Child Abuse, Sexual—
therapy. 3. Adolescent. 4. Child. 5. Prostitution—psychology. 6.
Psychotherapy—methods. WS 350.2 P3585y 2009]
  RC560.C46P43 2009
    362.76—dc22
                          2009002267

ISBN10: 0-415-40716-8 (pbk)
ISBN10: 0-415-40715-X (hbk)
ISBN10: 0-203-87418-8 (ebk)

ISBN13: 978-0-415-40716-8 (pbk)
ISBN13: 978-0-415-40715-1 (hbk)
ISBN13: 978-0-203-87418-9 (ebk)

Contents

Acknowledgements

This book would not have been possible without the inspiration from the young people I have met in my work. All have illustrated the complexities inherent within exploitative relationships. I dedicate this book to all young people, their friends, families and carers, who have suffered from sexual exploitation. I hope that the book will help to raise awareness of the damage that sexually exploitative relationships can cause.

One of the most important resources for young people who have experienced sexual exploitation is a sustained relationship with a practitioner. Indeed, many of the services have depended upon the determination and resilience of many workers who have struggled to keep their services going against all sorts of odds. They, with members of the National Working Group for Sexually Exploited Children and Young People (NWG) have, as friends and colleagues, informed and developed my thinking.

In particular, Nasima Patel alongside Mandy John-Baptitse have been with me from the start, with clarity in thinking and helpful insistence that child protection remain high on every agenda. Sheila Taylor has, with the motto 'where there is a will there's a way', shown the importance of keeping sexual exploitation in the thinking of all child care policy and practice service providers. Marilyn Haughton has always upheld the importance of the voice of the child with a sense of humour second to none. She has shown me how education can be taken to young people who have been excluded and abandoned. Ann Lucas has demonstrated how change can be brought about within statutory services while working in partnership with NGOs and Julie Harris and Paula Skidmore have maintained the importance of good, thorough academic scrutiny, reaching out to research difficult topics with a calm, sensitive and imaginative approach. Jo Phoenix has been a consistent strength, always achieving the daunting challenge of translating theory into practice, helping maintain a focus on the young person's self determination and agency. Sue Jago who suggested the subtitle for this book, has helped me to understand how policy can be developed through a relationship between young people and the work carried out by their practitioners.. Debbie Walmsley has, with her calm and thoughtful insight, continued to play an essential role with Comic Relief in developing and supporting this area of work. Mandy MacDonald, Wendy

Sheppard and Sara Swann who have been, with Tink Palmer, pioneers for this work; Irene Iveson, who raised awareness of parents and families needs after the tragic murder of her 17 year old daughter; Aravinda Kosaraju from Coalition Against Removal of Pimping (CROP); Camille Warrington and Nancy Purdy; Charlie Hedges, whose work on missing children has been so important. All have helped to raise the profile of the needs of sexually exploited children and young people through their work.

The book draws heavily on research work I carried out with Mary Williams and Christine Galvin in 2002 funded by the Joseph Rowntree Foundation (JRF) and Middlesex University. Charlie Lloyd from the JRF provided support and encouragement for the work to be completed. Throughout all of my work in this area, Professor Susanne MacGregor has been there as a mentor and role model. Her leadership in academic settings, in social policy, her thought and care on all areas of work that she is involved with have been an inspiration.

I want to say a particular thank you to colleagues at Bedfordshire University: David Barrett, John Pitts and Margaret Melrose have been central to the development of my work. Their writing, friendship, and critical appraisal of my work has, with others from the department and faculty at Bedfordshire led by Ravi Kohli and Michael Preston-Shoot respectively and administered by Cara Senouni, developed one of the best team of colleagues that I have had the privilege of working with. The editorial team at Routledge have supported me through the process of writing and editing the work.

I thank my family, including my two daughters who have patiently supported me throughout with laughter and without complaint, despite the odd comment about a school lunch box with a mouldy bread sandwich! They have encouraged my work through every step of the way. Finally, I want to thank my partner, John who has been a listening ear and critical reader. His support has been invaluable.

Introduction

Child sexual exploitation: Interconnected themes

This book focuses on the sexual exploitation of children and young people. It pulls together various strands of work that have taken place in the field and places the needs of the child at the centre. I will now outline some reoccurring and interconnected themes within the book. Firstly, the needs of individual children have to be seen within the context within which they live. The issue is that if we focus only on the needs of the individual young person, we thereby pathologise them. The social structure and circumstances that might have contributed to producing some of the young person's problems in the first place remain intact while the individual is seen as the problem. I hope to have incorporated the need to address the range of social inequalities that contribute to young people becoming vulnerable to sexual exploitation alongside looking at individual need.

This raises questions about the 'cause' of sexual exploitation. Some will argue that it is a direct result of a patriarchal system that creates gender power imbalances. To tackle sexual exploitation we need to focus on male sexual and physical violence towards women. While I have sympathy with this position, I explore some other, wider causes for sexual exploitation within the book, which put forward other viewpoints, and which address the needs of boys and young men alongside girls and young women. I hope to embrace a range of reasons for vulnerability to sexual exploitation, including economic inequality; familial problems such as drug and alcohol dependency and mental health problems; problems experienced by young people looked after and in care with the local authority; and individual problems such as low self-esteem, self-harming behaviour and problems with attachment.

Related to this I have argued that sexual exploitation is, as a form of sexual abuse, a concern for child protection. However, other agencies such as health and education within children's services have a central role in identifying and responding to sexually exploited children and young people. Child protection services have been developed primarily with the needs of children suffering from familial sexual abuse within the home in mind. They may not be adequately resourced to respond to the various needs of an older young person undergoing the transition to adulthood. This is a particularly pertinent point for young people between the ages of 16 and 18.

I also note that government guidance documents and different levels of legislation cannot be enough to protect the young people concerned. Through the updating of the Sexual Offences Act 1956 to the Sexual Offences Act 2003 we have a plethora of new legislation aimed at protecting children and young people from sexual exploitation, whether actual or intended. Children and young people are to be protected by law from non-consensual sexual activity (Sections 3 and 4) and from someone over 18 causing or inciting a child under 16 to engage in sexual activity (Section 10). The arranging or facilitating the commission of a child is a sexual offence, with the intent being an offence whether or not the sex takes place (Section 14), and meeting a child following grooming is an offence, again even if the intended sexual activity does not take place (Section 15) (Sexual Offences Act 2003).

However, this, along with the different policy guidance documents issued by the government on work with young people will not impact on sexually exploited young people unless they are implemented, their use reviewed, monitored and evaluated. I am aware that such call for evaluation is resource intensive, and I do not advocate that a call for data collection and monitoring of services is made without additional resourcing to support this. The point is that we need to know how many sexually exploited young people there are in the UK. We need to know what services exist to support them and learn from the lessons that they can teach us. Children's charities have taken a big step forward in guiding how this can happen (see Scott and Skidmore 2006 for an example). However, for health services (including sexual and mental health services), education and employment and police interventions to be effective, implementation strategies and evaluations are essential. This is particularly pertinent as the government has just issued its revised guidance on safeguarding sexually exploited children and young people (DCSF 2009). This is a step forward, but will only be effective if accompanied by an implementation strategy that aims to share examples of good practice across and between agencies in the country.

The book also touches on the familiar debate about whether the resources that are available for young people should be generic – tailored for universal use, or targeted – tailored for use by those most in need. The argument for universal services is that disadvantaged young people do not become stigmatised or labelled. All young people are encouraged to access the same level of service provision. The problem with this is that those who are most in need of service provision, the most alienated and disadvantaged, may not be able to access the service, or, if they do, may have to be excluded for fear of disrupting the majority. The argument for targeted services is based on the premise that a minority of young people have specific needs that require particular interventions with specially trained and supported staff. The recent focus on this debate is explored in a paper on 'Integrated Youth Support Services', which argues that while targeted youth support is about helping vulnerable young people with complex needs to access the intensive support they require, integrated youth support services are to 'provide services to *all* young people according to their needs' (Weinstock 2007: 1).

In this book I argue that while the focus should be on protecting sexually exploited children and young people from abuse through specialist targeted child protection interventions and safeguarding children boards, the generic universal providers should also be providing support services to encourage and enable all young people to access their service. Just as other young people, those who are sexually exploited will have, or will have had, aspirations to achieve their aims and dreams. As said by one young woman who, with support from a specialist project was reflecting on her situation:

> I don't want to be a junkie ... I should be living a very good life. The way I used to dream when I was a little girl. This is not my dream. This is not my dream at all. Its my nightmare. The worst nightmare
>
> (Issy, aged 17, in Pearce et al 2002)

Another, who following intense support from a targeted service provider, was able to engage with the universal provision, the local college noted that:

> In college you see a lot of young kids smiling. Why can't I be like that? Its about time I put my life together. I've learnt my mistakes with boys and everything. I'm not getting involved with a boy again. I'm going to concentrate on my studies and become someone someday.
>
> (Fi, aged 16, in Pearce et al 2002)

This young person was supported by both the targeted specialist project worker and by the college counselling support service to enable her to integrate into college life. This would not have been achieved without both of these services working together, alongside each other.

Finally, a theme that continues through the book is the importance of recognising the young person's own sense of agency. As reviews of practice and research have shown, many of these young people do not ask to be protected (Chase and Statham 2005). They may openly rebel against being seen as a victim, not wanting to identify with a child protection service but wanting to integrate into mainstream activities. As noted by a recent evaluation of services:

> All these young people present three major challenges to services attempting to intervene in their lives. First, they do not acknowledge their own exploitation. Second, they are extremely 'needy' for attention, 'love' and of belonging somewhere – and are reliant on abusive adults to meet these needs. Third, they have little previous experience of adult support and believe they are better off looking after themselves rather than relying on parents or professionals.
>
> (Scott and Skidmore 2006: 3)

Throughout the book I express a worry that an uncritical acceptance of the definition of the child as a victim of abuse can undermine the development of the same child's sense of agency. Many might be making choices, albeit limited choices (see Chase and Statham 2005 for more information on this) to cope with poverty and social exclusion. There has been a considerable drive to identify and address child poverty and the disadvantage that accompanies it (HM Treasury 2008). In 1999 the government made a pledge to end child poverty within a generation – by 2020. The first target to lift one million children out of poverty was missed by 300,000. To meet the 2010 target, the number of children in poverty must fall to 1.7 million. It is currently at 2.9 million (before housing costs) (HM Treasury 2008). Indeed, the Treasury noted that:

> Many people believe there is very little child poverty in the UK today. This is not the case: over a fifth of children are in poverty. The Government believes it is one of the most corrosive social issues facing the country, and it touches each and every person, indirectly if not directly. Child poverty is everyone's problem, and tackling it needs to be everyone's business.
>
> (HM Treasury 2008: 6)

And:

> Local authorities have a critical role in helping to eradicate child poverty by leading local action, engaging with and harnessing the resources of local communities to increase employment opportunities for all, preventing those at risk from falling into poverty and improving the life chances of young people.
>
> (HM Treasury 2008: 3)

As argued by a Joseph Rowntree Foundation study on poverty and exclusion, the:

> Government will need to extend its policy of increasing redistribution to low-income families [and] long-term policies working in this direction include better education and training for disadvantaged groups.
>
> (JRF 2006: 1)

Although not all sexually exploited children and young people come from situations of poverty and deprivation, research has shown that many do. In each of the chapters of the book I try to retain sight of how this, and the other different themes identified above are interconnected and experienced by the children and young people concerned.

Chapter outline

I have divided the book into two parts. Part 1 focuses on the policy context for work with sexually exploited children and young people while Part 2 identifies issues for practice. Although aspects of both policy and practice become entwined throughout, I have tried to clarify the context within which sexual exploitation sits in Part 1, and some of the issues faced by practitioners working with the young people concerned in Part 2.

PART 1

Chapter 1: Sexual exploitation: Child prostitution or child protection?

Chapter 1 explores the historical context within which sexual exploitation is located. It unpicks the developing discourse of sexual exploitation, identifying how it arose from discourses of child prostitution.

Chapter 2: Current policy and practice: Achievements and limitations

Chapter 2 looks more closely at the current policy framework within the UK, identifying the range of interventions that could be used to support sexually exploited children and young people and disrupt and prosecute those who abuse them.

Chapter 3: The trafficking of children and young people: Implications for work with sexually exploited children and young people

Chapter 3 considers the recent focus on the needs of trafficked young people. The trafficking of human beings, and in particular of children for the purpose of sexual exploitation, has raised significant concern, particularly in the last five years. The chapter clarifies some of the issues about identifying trafficked young people, defining them as trafficked, clarifying the different forms of trafficking (particularly the difference between international and trafficking of UK nationals within the UK). It argues for a child-centred perspective to dominate service delivery in this field.

Chapter 4: Adolescents in violent partnerships (AVP): Child abuse and domestic violence?

Chapter 4 addresses the contribution that work with adults who have experienced domestic violence can make to work with sexually exploited children and young people. With a particular focus on the older young people, those between 16 and 18 years of age, the chapter looks at the need to understand the nature of violence experienced by young people who might be in love with their abuser. It looks at the time that it takes for a victim of interpersonal violence to leave the perpetrator and at the different support systems that have been developed through work with victims of domestic violence (such as supported housing). These forms of intervention could usefully be applied to young people who are experiencing exploitative and violent interpersonal relationships. This recognises that children's services child protection agencies cannot be seen as the only resource with responsibility to support the young person away from violence and abuse.

PART 2

Chapter 5: Risk and resilience

Chapter 5 explores the different meanings of risk and resilience, looking at the application of both to sexually exploited children and young people. While it advocates the importance of identifying and challenging the risk factors that both push and pull young people into exploitative situations, it argues that a similar 'eye' needs to be held on the need to support the development of the young person's resilience. Seeing risk and resilience as a pair in partnership, the chapter advocates a range of interventions to support young people from different service providers.

Chapter 6: Doing research in the field of sexual exploitation

Chapter 6 looks at how research has both arisen from and informed discourses, policies and practice pertaining to sexual exploitation. It explores some of the gaps in research with this group of young people. Central to this is the relationship between research and practice and the need for emotional support for researchers undertaking the work. The chapter considers the ethical issues involved with undertaking research with this 'hard to reach' group and argues for supported, partnership research that uses gatekeepers appropriately and sensitively to access young people.

Chapter 7: Young people's participation

Young people's participation in the development and governance of youth services has become an important consideration in policy and practice. This chapter explores some of the complexities involved in accessing young people who might want to participate at this level, in supporting them to participate and in making the participation meaningful and worthwhile for them. Identifying a range of different activities through which the young person's voice can be heard, it argues that participation can have important benefits and outcomes for the young people concerned.

Chapter 8: Therapeutic outreach

Finally, this chapter explores the therapeutic needs of sexually exploited children and young people. It argues that many universal and targeted services, such as Child and Adolescent Mental Health Services (CAMHS) providers are poorly equipped to identify and respond to the number of mental health problems presented by many sexually exploited young people. Although there are some examples of good multi-agency work and supportive interventions, the therapeutic needs of the young people can often be overlooked. The chapter argues for a better awareness of the therapeutic needs of the young people, of the support structures that are needed for the staff working with them and for better integration of mental health interventions within generic service providers.

Key issues for practice

In summary, the book calls for 'sustained safeguarding': for the need to safeguard sexually exploited children and young people throughout the trajectory of exploitation. That is, at the early stages where preventative interventions can divert the young people from dangerous situations, through to the point where a young person is entrenched within an exploitative relationship or within behaviours that continue to put them at risk. At all stages of this sustained safeguarding, the young person should be worked with as a victim of abuse, not as a perpetrator of crime. The focus on sustained safeguarding means identifying and using resources to support 16 to 18 year olds as well as younger children. It should ensure that the needs of all young people are held with equal importance within the safeguarding agenda.

It also notes the need for 'Time aware', 'Relationship-based thinking' behind all interventions with sexually exploited children and young people. This recognises that young people will need time to build trusting and meaningful relationships with their practitioners. Change in the young person's circumstances will not happen overnight, but their situation could be aggravated by interventions that expect sudden, visible results. Similarly, the relationship-based thinking approach argues that staff themselves must be supported to manage the difficult and challenging behaviours presented by the young people.

Finally, the book calls for an investment in 'Therapeutic Outreach'. This recognises that staff need support to reach out to young people and to 'hold them in mind' even if they run from home or repeatedly go missing. This recognises that their difficult, rejecting and often aggressive behaviour is a sign of their distress. It also appreciates that the most damaged and disaffected sexually exploited young people will be unlikely to make and keep appointments at centre-based services. These young people will need support through outreach services that bear their therapeutic needs in mind.

In summary

Services for sexually exploited children and young people have developed over the last decade, with Children's Charities and some local authorities taking a lead in illustrating examples of good practice. Many inspired and enlightening lessons have been learned from this work. Unfortunately however, these examples are too few and far between. Many sexually exploited children and young people continue to have their needs unidentified and unmet. This means that those who intend to exploit them continue without redress. This must not continue. Too many children and young people have already died or had their lives damaged through sexual exploitation. To protect and safeguard children and young people from this abuse, we need to enable all local authorities across the country to address the sexual exploitation of children and young people through universal and targeted services. Otherwise we let down young people such as Jane, aged 17. Jane contacted the police after having been abducted, raped and sexually exploited by the man she called her boyfriend:

> you just feel like exploding and you just can't take no more regardless of what anyone is telling you to do. I just wanted to get out of there.
> That day when I finally phoned the police I felt so relieved. I would say that was definitely the happiest day of my life. I've actually done something.
>
> (Jane, in Pearce et al 2002)

Part 1

1 Sexual exploitation: Child prostitution or child protection?

In much of the reform rhetoric, the young prostitutes are portrayed as sexually innocent, passive victims of individual evil men. This imagery of individual sin, with its corresponding possibility of individual redemption, may have been comforting to these late – Victorian middle class reformers because it did not threaten the images of womanhood, childhood, and family life that had formed an essential part of their world view

(Gorham 1978: 355)

Introduction

The observation made by Gorham in 1978 above identifies some of the tensions that did, and still do, exist in discourses about child prostitution and sexual exploitation. Is the young person a passive 'innocent' victim, separated by the abuse they receive from 'normal' family lives? Indeed, the dominant perspective of the 1800s was of child prostitution as a 'veritable slave trade', where children are:

> snared, trapped and outraged either when under the influence of drugs or after a prolonged struggle in a locked room

These words, written in 1885, came from Stead, a journalist with a mission to protect girls from prostitution (see Gorham 1978: 353). The extract from the Pall Mall Gazette was his most 'successful story ever' and contributed to the drive for changes within The Criminal Law amendment Act of 1885, commonly known as Stead's Act, raising the age of consent to 16 years.

With such attention at that time, why do we, now, more than one hundred years later, still look at the sexual exploitation of children and young people as though it is a new problem? How can it be that some areas in the country are still confused about whether they should refer to child prostitution or child sexual exploitation, questioning what both mean or whether such things take place in their area? Why do we still have local authorities without procedures to guide their responses, relying on one or two isolated 'individuals with a mission' to raise attention about the problems (Jago and Pearce 2008)? Going back to the language used by Stead above, why did we then and do we continue to rely on sensationalist journalism pleading to audiences' hearts for the plights of individual young women, looking at the one-off individual cases without addressing the political context: the structural, social and economic circumstances of the young people as part of the picture?

In this chapter I explore some of these questions, looking at the changing perceptions and regulations of sexual exploitation, considering the policy and practice context within which it sits. As discourses of prostitution have changed and developed over the years, so too have perceptions of the role of women, sexuality and children's sexual exploitation (Self 2003, Phoenix and Oerton 2005). It is these that I explore below, leaving us with a better understanding of the tensions and difficulties facing practitioners working with individual young women and young men in the current context of safeguarding children.

Child prostitution: Repent or be dammed!

Stead attracted intense interest in child prostitution during his time. Indeed it is claimed that he 'subsequently served as a model for personalized and sensationalized form of muckraking that has become a permanent form of modern journalism' (Gorham 1978: 353). This prediction might well be seen to have been accurate, as similar sensationalised imagery and wording continues to provoke general interest in the twenty-first century. This 'social evil' that the newspaper was about to reveal in 1885 was the widespread existence of juvenile prostitution in London and the presence of an organised traffic in young English girls that supplied brothels on the continent. As with the modern awareness of debt bondage, concern was about a system of debt used against the girls who were imprisoned against their will. By 1884 Judith Butler, Bramwell Booth of the Salvation Army and other reformers were convinced that child prostitution was a problem for the country. In particular, they were concerned with finding a number of London brothels supplying young girls to upper class clientele.

What is of interest here is the difficulty that reformers of the 1880s had in distinguishing between their desire to both protect girls, the object of their concern, and their need to control them. Firstly, on the one hand, there is the aim to rescue and care for the innocent girl, whilst on the other hand there is the outrage, followed by the penalising, of the wayward immorality of sexually active young women (Self 2003). Gorham notes the inherent contradictions in the Victorian era between rescuing the deserving poor from destitution on the one hand, and penalising the 'promiscuous' undeserving reoffender on the other. She notes that the desire to rescue girls, who were, in almost all cases, young working class children, was influenced by whether the girls conformed to sexual stereotypes.

Although many progressive developments have been made in our generic understanding of young people's sexuality (Moore and Rosenthal 1992, 2006), and our specific understanding of child sexual exploitation (Chase and Statham 2005), the tension between care and control is as pertinent now as it was then (Phoenix 2002). The government guidance issued to local authorities in 2000 'Safeguarding Children Involved in Prostitution' and revived in 2009 proposes that the young people concerned are, first and foremost, to be worked with as victims of child abuse, with interventions directed through welfare agencies. However, for those young people who reject support and who 'persistently and voluntarily return' to selling sex, the criminal justice system is to intervene (DH 2000: 27; DCSF 2009).

The guidance argued that:

> it would be wrong to say that a boy or girl under 18 never freely chooses to continue to solicit, loiter or importune in a public place for the purpose of prostitution, and does not knowingly and willingly break the law … .persistence is generally understood in law to require a determined repetition of an activity
>
> (DH 2000: 27–28)

This threat of a shift from a caring response to compliant behaviour, to penalising challenging behaviour is one echoed in a number of child care policies since 2000. For example, the underpinning hypothesis of the 'respect agenda' of 2006 is that all young people, irrespective of race, gender, ability or economic circumstances are to be given access to opportunities to achieve well-being within the market economy (HO 2006a). Chapters 1 to 6 of the agenda outline a range of support for young people giving them opportunities to achieve in a number of ways in line with the five outcomes of 'Every Child Matters' (DfES 2004a). Chapters 7 and 8 on the other hand, outline a range of punitive interventions targeted at young people who challenge this or disrupt their own progress in accessing and using these opportunities.

Similarly, the green paper 'Youth Matters' laudably claims that 'we will ensure that young people with more serious problems receive an integrative package of support from someone they know and trust' (DfES 2005: 2). However, it also advocates withholding rewards from those young people who demonstrate antisocial behaviour. The meaning behind the language is clear: only those who behave will receive support and encouragement. New opportunities (through the use of opportunity cards) will be available to all young people:

> Except where they become involved in unacceptable or anti-social behaviour. In this case opportunity cards would be suspended or withdrawn
>
> (DfES 2005: para 94)

> poor behaviour is not acceptable
>
> (DfES 2005: para 80)

Sanctions should be used in response to any breaches

(DfES 2005: para 89)

And:

> increased opportunities do not come for free ... we therefore expect young people to respect the opportunities made available to them ... we will therefore not top up the opportunity cards of young people engaging in unacceptable behaviour ... In these circumstances, we believe that local authorities should withdraw or suspend use of the card
>
> (DfES 2005: para 116)

Previous experiences of abuse or relationship breakdowns may mean that the young person finds it extremely difficult to build a trusting and respecting relationship with an adult. If they also have experienced extreme poverty and deprivation in their local area, they may well be cynical about the value of an opportunity card. Disruptive behaviour is often demonstrative of frustration and anger experienced by young people who are growing into adulthood with limited resources and support (Pitts 2008). They may have learnt to feel resentful or suspicious of offers of support, continuing to reject help as a means of exerting some control over a life that might feel chaotic (Howe 1998: see Chapter 7 for more details on this topic).

The concern, a legacy remaining from the Victorian era referred to by Gorham, is whether the most damaged children and young people (indeed, the ones who are invariably demonstrating antisocial behaviour) are actually in a position to start to take responsibility for their actions. There is no doubt that many sexually exploited children and young people are difficult, challenging and hard to engage. Many may be rude, aggressive and caught in a cycle of running from home and engaging with informal economies (Scott and Harper 2006, Scott and Skidmore 2006, Pearce 2007b). The research in the field suggests that those who are the most challenging, the most difficult to engage are the ones who do persistently return to swapping or selling sex. They are unlikely to be able to make informed decisions about controlling their behaviour. They are the most disadvantaged, the most damaged and the most in need of welfare support. The results of a two-year evaluation of Barnardos services providing for sexually exploited children and young people showed a full spectrum of disadvantage experienced by the young people concerned. Of 42 of the young people using 10 Barnardos services, 19 had spent some part of their childhood in the looked after system, only four had no apparent history of abuse or neglect, almost all had disengaged from school in their early teens, 63% went missing from home at the initial assessment prior to referral to the project, one-third of these going missing for prolonged periods of time (Scott and Skidmore 2006: 43). Of a study of 55 young people, the 21 who were persistently selling sex were the most alienated from services, the most difficult to engage and carried the largest number of problems at any one time (Pearce et al 2002).

These young people faced a range of problems, often compounded by the influence of a manipulative abusive adult. If the young persons' antisocial or rejecting behaviour becomes the focus of attention, their social, economic and personal vulnerabilities are overshadowed as they are 'blamed' for their actions. There is increasing concern amongst many social researchers that the focus on young people's antisocial behaviour develops a 'blame' culture, shifting attention onto the individual child's behaviour and away from the social, moral and economic context they find themselves in.

> There has been too much emphasis on anti-social behaviour and too ready willingness to attribute blame either to parents or to young people themselves
>
> (Coleman and Scofield 2007: xi)

As with the nineteenth and twentieth centuries, we, in the twenty-first century continue to respond to the behaviour of the exploited rather than challenge the overall context within which the exploitation occurs, penalising those who reject welfare interventions.

Gorham goes onto highlight how many of the girls engaged in prostitution were not passive, sexually innocent victims but were responding to situations of limited choice. The 'causes of juvenile prostitution were to be found in an exploitative economic structure' (Gorham 1978: 355). This is endorsed by Judith Walkowitz who argued that many working class young women in late-Victorian England had few other ways of earning money to survive (Walkowitz 1992). A critique that fully recognised these economic realities would have demanded a much more radical transformation of the structure of society than was implied by the reformers' programme of individual moral uplift. Gorham shows that emerging concepts of childhood were influenced by class divisions as the middle and upper classes started to have time and money to dedicate to their children's welfare, whilst working classes did not. Working class children became separated from their parents at a much earlier age than did their middle and upper class counterparts, often needing to be self-supporting by 13 years old. The respectable working class girls went into service while the 'rough' and 'outcast' working class girls started work earlier in more manual labour. For example, agricultural girls worked in agricultural gangs and:

> in London the girl children of the poorest or 'outcast' class faced conditions that do much to explain the prevalence of juvenile prostitution ... There was a chronic oversupply of girls for a limited amount of ill-paid work ... it was the brutal bleakness of their lives that probably led many young girls into prostitution. The money and the 'gay' life must have seemed very attractive to a fur puller who made a few shillings a week or a domestic servant who had to sleep in a damp basement kitchen
>
> (Gorham 1978: 373–374)

What can we learn from looking back to this time? There are some reoccurring questions arising from this historical legacy of debates around child prostitution and child sexual exploitation here. The question of the young person's agency arises as we consider if the young person is making their own decision (albeit one in circumstances of constrained choice – see Chase and Statham 2005) to sell sex as a means of coping with poverty. Are they a passive victim to be supported through welfare-based interventions or are they to be punished or 'treated' for transgressing legal and moral codes? Is the transgression to be understood as a 'rational', 'normal' response to abnormal circumstances such as extreme poverty or previous experience of abuse? How does poverty and deprivation impact on the young person's vulnerability to abuse from exploitative adults involved in informal economies?

With these questions in mind, I look now at the more recent changes and developments in policy and practice guidance for work with young people, noting the shift in language from young people involved in prostitution to sexually exploited children and young people.

Social welfare approaches: Sexual abuse and social exclusion

Sexual abuse

The inter-world war period saw the emergence of feminist and child welfare organisations seeking to explain the sexual precociousness in girls as an outcome of sexual abuse (Brown A. 2004: 349). Despite the resulting focus on the abusive adult, Brown explores the continued tensions around proportioning blame on the child. She refers to the conflict between two key organisations developed to address child abuse: the Association for Moral and Social Hygiene (AMSH) and the National Vigilance Associate (NVA). The AMSH emphasised the promiscuity, and therefore the blame of girls aged 14 and 15; and the latter emphasised the abuse, and therefore the abstention from blame, of pre-pubescent children.

These two approaches highlighted the confused approaches that were emerging in studies of adolescence as a developmental life stage and to the sliding scale of awareness of sexual abuse: with 'the helpless innocent child at the one end of the scale and the precocious temptress at the other' (Justice of the Peace 1925 in Brown A. 2004: 350). This confusion pivots around questions of when childhood finishes and adulthood begins: when interventions shift from protecting the innocent child to holding the adult responsible for their actions. As explored by Coleman and Hendry, the nature of adolescence is the transitional process involved for the young person changing both physically and psychologically from child to adult (Coleman and Hendry 1999). During such transition, both the young person and the adults responding to them can be confused about where the young person sits on this developmental continuum.

The confusion is apparent in the The Street Offences Act 1959 which gave no age distinction to the term 'common prostitute' or to soliciting offences. More recently, the Government Prostitution Strategy (HO 2006b) has been criticised for confusing issues relating to adult women with child protection issues facing young people. The strategy makes a number of important and helpful interventions in work with children and young people. However, Brooks-Gordon argues that children and adults are conflated within the strategy, women being portrayed solely as victims of abuse through prostitution (and therefore infantile) rather than independent agents making their own decisions about their work (Brooks-Gordon 2006: 60). By still allowing for conviction for offences relating to prostitution, children are given adult status as offenders responsible for their actions.

Social exclusion

It was not until the rapid development of the welfare state following the Second World War that an emergence of left wing radicalism within some parts of the increasingly professional welfare services challenged an approach that focused on individual situations of child abuse. In particular, perspectives that aimed to address young people's experiences of class and gender power dynamics, began to come to the fore.

The 1960s, 70s and early to mid 80s saw the comprehensive school system making attempts to engage with working class cultures while the radical social work tradition was challenging social workers to consider the impact of social class on their client groups. These approaches placed a particular focus on engaging with the social, economic and political structures that played a part in service users' conditions and circumstances (Bailey and Blake 1975, Langan and Lee 1989). Classic texts such as Paul Willis's 'Learning to labour: how working class kids get working class jobs' (Willis 1977) and Sue Sharpes's 'Just like a girl' (Sharpe 1977) looked critically at how young people from working class cultures responded to the dominant values of the education system, while other more generic studies focused on the role of young people from working class cultures within the labour market of the time (Clarke et al 1979). At the same time, questions about the value of multicultural approaches to service provision were raised, asking for an enhanced awareness of the pressures on young people resulting from racism. This focused both on service delivery and on young people's potential to access services (Amos and Parmar 1981, Gilroy 1987). Later a plethora of work developed, focusing a critical eye on the social construction of girls' and young women's sexuality, their academic achievements and of the gendered and racialised nature of the public and private worlds of work and home (see McRobbie 1991 and Mirza 1992 for further work in this area).

Similarly, critical voices were asking questions within social work and youth justice (then intermediate treatment) about the apparent gendered distinctions between 'bad' boys and 'mad' girls within social care networks. The high numbers of 'mad' young women being referred for psychiatric assessment and being received into care for being 'in moral danger' and 'beyond control' were contrasted against the high numbers of 'bad' young men, committing offences and being worked with by the youth justice system. Researchers and practitioners were beginning to question the way that gendered stereotypes were being acted out by the young people on the one hand and endorsed through practitioner and policy interventions on the other (Hudson 1988). Although the involvement of young people in prostitution was not the centre of attention, the gendered definition of 'in moral danger' was being questioned.

Although increasingly being criticised as the antics of the 'looney left', these developments meant three things. Firstly, they shifted the focus from individual pathology to structural inequality, looking at the economic and social conditions of many working class families. Secondly, they raised questions about the gendered and racialised nature of adolescence and sexual identity, both in the young persons' expression of sexuality and in the ways that this is controlled through welfare interventions. Finally, they laid the ground for an awareness of the impact of exclusion from school, from mainstream health provisions and from youth work services. The developing discourses around social exclusion tried to address the inherent inequalities within isolated and specific geographical and social communities (Skelton and Valentine 1998) and to reverse the impact of cycles of deprivation, brought about, in part, by the labelling of individual young people and the communities that they occupied as deprived and disadvantaged. Worryingly, this has more recently been turned into a blame culture which can pinpoint an irresponsible antisocial 'underclass' as the cause of all social problems (Gillies 2000).

This focus on the relationship between structural, cultural and individual factors influencing the behaviour on young people was important. Shildrick and MacDonald (2008: 45) continue to explore the relationship between 'individual agency, local (sub) cultures and the social structural context'. They argue that the three issues have each to be worked with together. Therefore, we need to address the young persons' own sense of agency, their peer and family or care groupings and the social and economic context within which they function when developing these specialist services.

Concern has been expressed that while service delivery is seen to be a problem of the individual, or of the individual and their immediate family under the jurisdiction of child protection and safeguarding boards, the important consideration of the young persons' peer and social groupings and socio-economic environment may be overlooked. In other words, an onus on child protection can mean that the work with the individual takes place without due regard to the context within which they live. But, poverty and social exclusion are complex issues, well established in debates about the sale of sex and exploitation of children for many generations (Pitts 1997, Barrett 1999, Phoenix 2002, Self 2003). Despite much debate, it has been a difficult one for policy makers to respond to appropriately. Essentially, changing economic and structural inequalities is a harder, lengthier job than trying to isolate a remedy for individual 'bad' behaviour. Without a sustained political drive to address the longer-term impact of poverty and disadvantage, policy makers and practitioners find themselves looking to work focusing on individual behaviour. This was seen in developments made to work with sexual exploitation during the 1990s and beyond.

From children involved in prostitution to child sexual exploitation

The 1990s saw a renewed focus on issues facing children involved in prostitution. It was during this time that language began to change from one using the term 'prostitution' to one that was focused on 'exploitation'. In 1995 the Children's Society produced an influential report titled 'The games up' which helped to raise attention to:

> the sexual exploitation of children and young people while encouraging a more constructive analysis of the factors that precipitate their involvement in prostitution.
>
> (Lee and O'Brien 1995: 3)

The report was important in that it managed to encourage awareness both of the individual needs of young people who were involved in prostitution and of the social and economic circumstances that they faced. Preempting the current awareness of 'constrained choice' (Chase and Statham 2005), the report noted that children involved in prostitution may create a version of reality that condones their use of the only power that they have left over themselves: the power to use or sell their body. Importantly, the report also identifies the high level of young people in care being involved in prostitution, noting in particular a correlation between experiences of residential care and coercion into prostitution. Children in care found that their access to health and education facilities was made harder by their lack of financial resources. They suffered from the:

> lack of access to the benefit system and housing, and their detachment from education, training and employment opportunities which is common amongst care leavers
>
> (Lee and O'Brien 1995: 13)

The report was most influential in its stark presentation of the high numbers of young people being punished through the criminal justice system for offences relating to prostitution, offences that the report claims to result from experiences of abuse, poverty and coercion. Between 1989 and 1993 a total of 1758 cautions and 1435 convictions were issued to young women under 18 years in England and Wales for prostitution-related offences. All but a few of the cautions, and all of the convictions used Section 1 of the Street Offences Act 1959 for soliciting and loitering. The same period saw 46 cautions issued to young men under 18 years for offences relating to their involvement in prostitution, 38 coming under the Sexual Offences Act 1956, the remainder coming under the Street Offences Act 1959. Forty-eight convictions were issued to young men for offences relating to soliciting. A deeper analysis of the figures showed that the number of cautions issued to young women aged 14 years increased more than two and a half times between 1989 and 1993 (Lee and O'Brien 1995: 40–47).

The report argued that there was no evidence to suggest that criminalising the young person acts as a deterrent from returning to selling sex. Few of the young people concerned felt that they have other choices for survival available to them. It also noted that the onus on criminalisation prevented young people from accessing support; while they were at risk of being criminalised, young people on the street were extremely unlikely to turn to the police for help to challenge those who were abusing them. Being unable to turn to the police, young people also felt alienated from social work providers who they felt to be inaccessible and unavailable. Indeed, with busy caseloads, the then social services departments were unlikely to view those involved in prostitution as high priority (Aldgate 1994 in Lee and O Brien 1995).

The report finishes with recommendations ranging from supporting families to reduce the prevalence of violence in the home: providing counselling to children and young people and addressing the lack of resources available to those working in residential care.

> It is known that poverty is a contributory factor to young people entering the care system in the first place yet the residential care system itself is chronically under-resourced
>
> (Lee and O'Brien 1995: 53)

It calls for awareness raising of the needs of homeless young people, for the development of further supported housing schemes for young people and for additional resources to support children and young people from poorer families and environments.

> the reinstatement of the right to benefit, or the meeting of the training guarantee with sufficient good quality and appropriate programs, would provide income for thousands of young people currently living in poverty
>
> (Lee and O'Brien 1995: 55)

This work was not taking place in isolation during the 1990s. An important literature review of young people involved in prostitution noted that the young people concerned experienced high levels of exclusion from school, from safe accommodation and from employment possibilities (Jesson 1993). Research was identifying the clear relationship between running from home and entering prostitution. As well as discussing a range of routes into prostitution, Barrett raised awareness of the dangers facing young people living on the street (Barrett 1997). Data from Centrepoint, which ran a London refuge for under 16 year olds, noted that of the young people using the resource, 39% had no money on them at all, a further 48% only having up to £39 to their name (Barter 1996: 47, Centrepoint 1997: 6). Increasing recognition was given to the impact of running from home, with estimations that within six weeks of running most young people will be drawn into using drugs and selling sex as coping mechanisms for survival (Kirby 1995, Pearce 1999, Green et al 1997). Questions about the impact of homelessness, problem drug use and exclusion from school on young people's propensity to sell or swap sex as a means of survival were being asked. These refocused the interest in appropriate support for these young people, highlighting the inadequacy of interventions through the criminal justice system.

While helpful in raising awareness of the impact of poverty and social deprivation on young people, this work also began a closer examination of how the young people began to sell sex. Working from the premise that no one wakes up one day and says 'I know, I will go out and sell sex', Barnardos took a lead in developing a model for the 'routes into prostitution' (Swann et al 1998). They developed a model for entry, now commonly called the 'grooming method'. Barnardos was developing a firm practice base in work with the young people concerned, taking a lead in providing support through specific dedicated workers who maintained outreach and centre-based activities for young people involved in prostitution. Specifically the 'Streets and Lanes Project' began to advocate further on the needs of the young people and were part of identifying the techniques used by abusers to entice and 'groom' young people into prostitution (for further details on the Streets and Lanes Barnardos Project and the grooming method, see www.barnardos.org.uk).

The 'grooming model for sexual exploitation', explained the process whereby an abusive adult entices a young person into becoming dependent upon them. Invariably, this involved the young person believing they are in love with their abuser. The pattern moves through a process where the abuser flatters the young person, giving them attention, accommodation and other gifts. The young person increasingly becomes dependent upon the abuser who invariably isolates them from family and friends and encourages them to become reliant upon drugs and alcohol. The young person is then forced or coerced into swapping or selling sex to raise money for the 'boyfriend'. This model is one that firmly incorporates exploitation as the central feature to child prostitution, and has been used as an argument to shift the language away from children involved in prostitution to child sexual exploitation:

> Barnardos had been a key player in raising awareness of sexual exploitation and developing an analysis of the nature of the problem over the previous decade. A high profile campaign of the late 1990s 'Whose Daughter Next?' (Barnardos 1998) had influenced government development of guidance on safeguarding children and young people abused through prostitution and identified them as victims of abuse rather than 'young prostitutes'
>
> (Scott and Harper 2006: 314)

This model, which has informed many of the child protection procedures in working with sexual exploitation, clearly shifts the identification of the child from being a perpetrator of crimes such as soliciting, to being a victim of abuse. However, there have been some criticisms that although appropriately explaining one route into sexual exploitation, the grooming model is only one of many ways in which a young person becomes exploited. A young person may not be in a particular relationship with one so-called 'boyfriend', but may be selling sex to a number of people as a means of getting money, drugs or alcohol (Phoenix 2002). If they are running from home, they might choose to take a bed for the night in exchange for some sexual activity. They may think that they can manage what is happening to them, or they may think that the exploitation is something that they will tolerate so that the relationship can continue and they can receive drugs, accommodation or other repayments that appear to be essential to their survival (Pearce et al 2002, Scott and Skidmore 2006). Indeed, as will be explored in Chapter 5, they may have built a resilience that enables them to tolerate their situation and, through weighing it up, decide that it is better than being on the run, homeless or without any money.

In other words, some, but not all, young people may end up swapping or selling sex because they are groomed and coerced. Others may feel that they are making their own decision about how to best survive their circumstances. More recently, it has become apparent that young people may be sexually exploited through use of the internet, through mobile phones or through processes of trafficking into and within the UK. The point here is that the work of the Children's Society, the NSPCC, Barnardos, and other important charities such as Centrepoint raised awareness of the risk factors that push certain young people into sexually exploitative situations, strengthening the argument for decriminalisation of these young people.

Changes in policing

These issues were taken up by the police who were in the forefront of having to address these contradictions. The Association of Chief Police Officers (ACPO) issued guidance on 'child prostitution' in 1998, noting that a) the Children's Society report 'The games up' highlighted the continued existence of child prostitution; and b) the Children Act 1989 called for the welfare of the child to be at the centre of all interventions. The ACPO guidance noted that statutory agencies, including the police, held a primary obligation to protect children in moral or physical danger and that they should be more actively pursuing those who abuse or coerce the children. The police formed a working group to address these issues. They agreed that ACPO should produce guidelines to be 'part of a genuine support and diversion program for young people caught up in prostitution' (Brain et al 1998: 3).

The resulting ACPO guidelines noted the need for young people to be removed to a place of safety as soon as identified as at risk of involvement in prostitution, and that they should then be referred to a multidisciplinary forum to assess their needs and circumstances rather than to be issued with a caution. The guidelines claimed that interviews with the child were to be conducted as though the child was a victim of abuse, rather than as a perpetrator of crimes associated with prostitution. The police should be involved in protecting the child during the lengthy stage of exiting from prostitution. However, the guidelines did not advocate decriminalising, retaining the powers to prosecute as a last resort following discussion with the multidisciplinary forum and the Crown Prosecution Service (Brain et al 1998).

A pilot scheme was established in Wolverhampton to pilot the guidelines and to focus on arrest and prosecution of abusers. Following the procedures outlined above, the pilot showed that during a seven-month period between 1997 and 1998, 43 children (between 11 and 17 years of age) entered the scheme, 11 worked with police as witnesses against their abusers, 21 cooperated with police but did not want to provide witness statements, and a further 11 were waiting to be fully investigated. In over 20 cases intervention prevented or disrupted children being sexually exploited, 9 adults were charged with serious criminal offences, 4 adults were in custody awaiting trail and 4 were on conditional bail, awaiting trial. Laying the foundations for the focus on multi-agency work of the government guidance on safeguarding children involved in prostitution, this pilot scheme was an essential part to beginning to change policy and practice (Brain et al 1998).

Conclusion

There has, and continues to be, confusion about how to work with young people who challenge the boundaries of expected sexual activity through adolescence (Moore and Rosenthal 2006). If the young people are using sexual activity for financial support, and are being aggressive, manipulative and rejecting in the process, it is hard to hold the image of them as victims of abuse. If, as will be explored further in Chapter 7, they are not only selling sex but are also challenging the gendered roles that are expected in heterosexual relationships outside the comfort of age-appropriate boundaries (a boy or girl selling sex to an older woman or older man for example) they are isolated away from the fundamental assumptions of 'healthy' adolescent development. However, a tolerance of unacceptable relationships is not the answer, as all children and young people, irrespective of the financial and social pressures they face, are entitled to a childhood and adolescence without abuse. Good practice in youth and social work teaches us that an uncritical collusion with the activities of young people who are testing boundaries for whatever the reason is not helpful (Crimmens et al 2005). If practice were to turn a blind eye to the exploitation that might be happening because the young person is saying that they 'want' an abusive relationship, it would be failing the child, failing to offer them the protection they are entitled to.

It is clear that there are some lingering problems for those developing policy and practice to protect and empower sexually exploited children and young people. These, in essence, centre on how services can be delivered to both support the individual young people concerned whilst addressing the deeply entrenched problems of abuse and violence in informal economies, some of which are developed primarily to meet the need of abusive adults, but others which evolve in response to poverty and long-term deprivation. While improved child protection policies and procedures can better support the individual young person, and improved policing and multi-agency work can result in more convictions of abusive adults, the deeper impact of the relationship between abuse and poverty, racism, gender power imbalances and social class will continue to create tension for many young people trying to achieve autonomous, independent status. I move now to looking at how more recent policy and practice has identified and worked with these issues.

2 Current policy and practice: Achievements and limitations

A recent OFSTED report indicates a clear link between the level of resources allocated to a service and the quality of its work ... The availability of well trained, high quality committed staff – youth workers who stay in post long enough to build the trusting relationships which young people value – is key to success. So too is funding which is sustained over time ...

... Regular participation throughout the teenage years is particularly important for the most disengaged and hard to reach young people for whom interventions need to be planned as medium or long term ...

(DCSF 2007: 28)

Introduction

The above comments from the government initiative 'Aim high for young people: a 10 year strategy for positive activities' (DCSF 2007) are just two of many which advocate funded opportunities for the most marginalised and disaffected young people within the UK. They reflect the need for long-term funding for the work. This has been identified by youth workers, researchers and specialist services in touch with sexually exploited children and young people, who have argued that effective work with sexually exploited children and young people is reliant upon specialist services being adequately funded, not for a one-year period but for the medium and long term, so that trusting relationships can be built and sustained (Melrose and Barrett 2004, Chase and Statham 2005, Scott and Skidmore 2006). Unfortunately, far too many of the few specialist services for sexually exploited children and young people that do currently exist in the UK have limited funding, often for one year only. As a result, they place substantial time and effort into trying to protect themselves from the regular threats to their continued existence. This does not provide a conducive environment for developing high-quality sustained interventions that the staff and young people can rely upon, and ultimately undermines the development and sharing of good practice.

Although the knowledge base and the policy framework for sexually exploited children and young people has improved since 2000, we still find ourselves in situations where most local authorities have few, if any, resources for follow-up work with some of the most damaged and marginalised sexually exploited children and young people in their locality. This chapter gives an overview of some of the developments that have taken place in policy and practice with sexually exploited children and young people since the issuing of the Department of Children Schools and Families (DCSF) guidance in 2000.

Safeguarding Children Involved in Prostitution (SCIP) Guidance: 2000 and beyond

By 2000, the need to understand sexually exploited children and young people as victims of abuse was enshrined within government guidance. The government's guidance for 'Safeguarding Children Involved in Prostitution' (SCIP guidance, DH 2000) firmly argued that the young people concerned were to be understood as victims of abuse from sexual exploitation. This SCIP guidance was a break-through as it stipulated that the then Social Services and Area Child Protection Committees (now Children's Services and Local Safeguarding Children Boards) had a responsibility for safeguarding children from exploitation. Area Child Protection Committees were advised to establish protocols, subcommittees and service delivery resources for protecting sexually exploited children and young people in their area.

The guidance notes that children involved in prostitution may not be visible to a casual or even to an informed observer:

> it is a 'hidden problem' and is a 'tragedy for any child' exposing them to abuse and assault, and may even threaten their lives. They can be robbed of their childhood, self esteem, opportunities for good health, education and training
>
> (DH 2000: 5)

I challenge the proposition that the problem is necessarily hidden later. For here, it is important that the government of the time recognised that sexual exploitation was not being identified and that children and young people were being harmed through this abuse. It noted that its purpose is to help agencies to recognise the problem and to 'treat the child primarily as a victim of abuse' (DH 2000: 5–6). The guidance provided helpful information about child protection procedures that should be enacted to protect a young person, about the range of agencies who should be involved (health, youth service and education for example) and about the legislation (now with an overdue need for updating in line with the Sexual Offences Act 2003) that could be used to disrupt and prosecute abusers. Although this was a great step forward, there continues to be a number of accompanying issues that are still being struggled with to date.

Variations in provision between local authorities

The guidance was just that: a document that outlined what local authorities 'should' do, issued without an implementation or reporting strategy, without a mechanism for data collection and without a process for annual review of progress. As a result, some local authorities do, to this day, remain without a working protocol to oversee provision and without a service to deliver support to the young people concerned. Nine years after the publication of the guidance, while most local authorities have been able to develop protocols, not all have local multi-agency subcommittees and even fewer have access to a dedicated service for the young people concerned (Jago and Pearce 2008). Although a cross-government, National Plan for Safeguarding Children from Commercial Sexual Exploitation was published in 2001 (DH/HO 2001), there has been little, if any, action to ensure that this is kept up to date and that departments are delivering on the commitments made. One of these commitments of the cross-government national plan was for it to be updated on an annual basis:

> The national plan is not a static document but will be developed on a year by year basis to ensure that it remains up-to-date and continues to focus on priorities for action. As in the development of the national plan itself, an inclusive approach will be pursued, drawing together expertise for across the voluntary sector, relevant professional bodies and government
>
> (DH/HO 2001: 3)

This annual review has not taken place, the implications of the national plan and the SCIP guidance being left without enforcement in many authorities. It is established that there is variation between local authorities' ability and willingness to deliver on central government initiatives. Local party politics and the history of governance within the authority all have a part to play in prioritising policy and putting it into practice (Jones and MacGregor 1998). Without a formal review of progress, many initiatives can remain sidelined or ignored. There has been one formal review of the progress of the use of the SCIP guidance. In 2002 the government commissioned Swann and Balding to undertake a review of its implementation. Here, Swann noted the background to her work with sexually exploited children and young people, highlighting her use of the Barnardos triangles as models for understanding and working with sexual exploitation. These triangles, taken to a world congress in 1994 and used in the Utting Report 'People like us' (Utting 1997), have provided a helpful framework for sexual exploitation interventions

The review undertaken by Swann and Balding was designed to look at the impact of the guidance on local authority service provision two years after its publication. It reviewed all 146 Area Child Protection Committees (ACPCs) in the country, and then carried out an in-depth survey of 50 ACPCs. Of all ACPCs in the country, 76% of local authorities said that they knew that

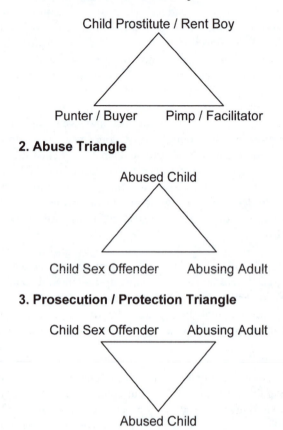

1. Prostitution / Sex Industry

Child Prostitute / Rent Boy

Punter / Buyer   Pimp / Facilitator

2. Abuse Triangle

Abused Child

Child Sex Offender   Abusing Adult

3. Prosecution / Protection Triangle

Child Sex Offender   Abusing Adult

Abused Child

Figure 2.1 A model for understanding abuse through prostitution. (Sara Swann)

there were children involved in prostitution in their area, 62% knowing of boys as well as girls involved. Sixty-five per cent said that they had protocols in action to cover work with children involved, leaving 35% without a protocol. Fifty-one per cent said that they had a subcommittee established to address the problem while only 30% were able to say that they had a specialist resource to support young people involved. Of the targeted survey of 50 ACPCs, 34% said they had no numerical data on how many times the protocol was used. Six per cent had young people on their subcommittee and 14% said that they started to work towards prosecuting abusers. Most importantly, only 6% said that they believed they were meeting the dual aim of protecting children and prosecuting abusers. This 2002 review showed that although the guidance was being used by 65% of the ACPCs to create protocols, only 30% had access to any specialist resource available to work with the young people concerned.

Without a requirement to record relevant data and to report on progress, many local areas have remained without a dedicated service and therefore without proactive work to identify and engage with young people. Protocols for protecting young people have little impact if they cannot ensure that the young person concerned is contacted, engaged with and supported: identification and engagement now known to be the first two essential components to an effective child exploitation strategy (Jago and Pearce 2008). The two aims of the SCIP guidance: protecting children and prosecuting abusers, both rely on effective identification of the young people concerned and engagement with them through relationship-based intervention (see Chapter 7). Efforts to prosecute abusers will be hindered if the young person is not being supported as a key witness. Such support cannot be a one-off meeting, but needs to be grounded in a strong relationship between key worker and young person in a trusted and established context. This will be able to support the young person through the trauma of giving evidence and taking the case through court. The support given to key witnesses by police, the Crown Prosecution Service (CPS) and the court processes is changing. However, no case will be without repercussions for the young person who has been a victim. Proper engagement with them through committed relationship-based interventions is, therefore, a central part to any child sexual exploitation strategy.

A sexual exploitation strategy

A recent review of some Local Safeguarding Children Boards' (LSCBs') capacity to disrupt and prosecute abusers has confirmed the range of different responses being made by local authorities to the problem of sexual exploitation in their area. Jago and Pearce (2008) sent out requests to the 144 safeguarding children boards in the country for information about strategies they employed for protecting sexually exploited children and young people, including those strategies targeted at disrupting and prosecuting abusers. Twenty LSCBs responded with positive actions to be included in the scoping exercise, 14 of whom had disruption and prosecution initiatives in protocols in place to address sexual exploitation (Jago and Pearce 2008: 10). Eight were undergoing a process to introduce new arrangements and six had dedicated operations in place at the time of the scoping exercise. Operations were taking place while the young people concerned were being supported in ongoing relationships with dedicated workers, the existence of a service to identify and engage the young people being a central feature to securing a successful operation.

The findings showed that in many areas there was evidence of a lack of focus on the proactive investigation of the perpetrators of child sexual exploitation, and that police child protection units had been traditionally reactive. However, the move to include the police child protection units within public protection units (PPUs) has helped to develop a more proactive approach (Jago and Pearce 2008: 12). In summary, it argues that a child sexual exploitation strategy must include four key ingredients. It must start with a process whereby sexually exploited children and young people are being *identified*. This means having training at a local level to help staff in universal service provision to be familiar with the early warning signs and key indicators. Then there must be an adequately resourced targeted, specialist provision that *engages* with the young person, providing support, ongoing one-to-one work and intensive intervention around the problems facing the young person. Thirdly, the strategy must include awareness of how to *disrupt* the actions of the abuser, disruption being a key element to protecting the child. In essence, disruption is not a 'soft option' (Jago and Pearce 2008: 22). Finally, the strategy needs to address the process of *prosecuting* the abuser, with joint work between police, dedicated specialist service providers, children service managers and use of the full wide range of legislation available. These four components: identification, engagement, disruption, and prosecution cannot work in isolation from each other. An effective strategy must include all four components. This has been recognised in the DCSF's new guidance for safeguarding sexually exploited children and young people brought into effect during 2009.

The Jago and Pearce (2008) scoping exercise identified a great range of levels of provision across the country. Exploring why certain areas had more established interventions to protect young people from sexual exploitation than others, it identified certain trigger factors that have helped, or prompted, a local authority to develop protocols and service provision. Sadly, one of the most significant motivators has been when the death of a child has been attributed to resulting from sexual exploitation. This has been behind some local authorities, such as Sheffield and Blackpool for example, setting up dedicated units, teams and services specifically for sexually exploited young people.

Another key motivating factor has been the presence of one of the national charities (mainly the Children's Society, Barnardos or National Society for the Prevention of Cruelty to Children; NSPCC) promoting the work in the area, often after having undertaken a scoping exercise to ascertain the scale of the problem. Also, the existence of a lone, local 'pioneer' in the authority, campaigning and advocating for sexually exploited children and young people has been a central drive to the establishment of a service.

The report explores the complex reasons that some local authority safeguarding boards have not been able to expose the realities within this 'hidden' problem of sexual exploitation. There is a genuine lack of knowledge and awareness of the nature and scale of sexual exploitation; of the way to respond if the stone is turned and cases are revealed; and a fear of the implications for resource allocation where services are already stretched. However, as is argued by Barnardos, longer-term savings can be made where early intervention is in place and practice across the country has shown that young people can be supported out of sexually exploitative situations and into employment, training and independent living if the specialist resources (advocated by the SCIP guidance 2009 and the National Plan 2001) are there to support them.

Sustained safeguarding

The problem remains, however, of how to enable all safeguarding boards and multi-agency service providers to prioritise the work and develop appropriate services. The new, updated SCIP government guidance 'Safeguarding children and young people from sexual exploitation' is, at this time, not supported by a government interdepartmental 'National Plan'. Neither is it supported by an implementation strategy with annual review on its effectiveness. It is possible that safeguarding boards, education, health and housing services will, by default, continue to vary in the extent that the new guidance is used and will default on the commitments required as they respond to other priorities. Sexual exploitation may continue to be marginalised as a problem of 'promiscuous' teenagers who, after a few years, will disappear as they mature and fall into the remit of adult services. The tragic case of Baby P, and the subsequent reviews focusing on the threshold for intervention with vulnerable young children, highlights the very real problem of training, resource allocation and questions about the threshold for intervention in child protection cases. While this is, at the moment, focused on safeguarding younger children, it is an ideal time for the question of developing sustained safeguarding, that is, safeguarding that continues through the transitional period of childhood into adolescence to adulthood. I advocate that one way of doing this is to put the aims of every child matters into effect. That is, to create multi-agency work that does not see the safeguarding of children and young people to be only the prerogative of child protection social workers.

Multi-agency service provision for sexually exploited children and young people

The guidance (DH 2009) notes the role that a range of service providers can play in safeguarding young people from sexual exploitation. However, the principle focus becomes one primarily concerned with child protection. I have argued elsewhere that although this is important, it is equally essential that all other services (education, health and housing, for example) are trained to identify problems of sexual exploitation, and to engage with the young people themselves, delivering a range of appropriate services to them (Pearce 2007b).

As noted above, The cross-government National Plan on Safeguarding Children from Commercial Sexual Exploitation (DH/HO 2001), set tasks for the range of different central and local government departments. However, this has, in the main been overlooked, poorly implemented and has not been reviewed on an annual basis to keep up to date with the changing policy context. As the policy context for work with young people has changed and become more complex, so too have the health provisions, educational contexts, employment opportunities and benefit allowances facing many adolescents. It is helpful to outline just some of these initiatives to highlight how they could work to support sexually exploited children and young people.

Every child matters: Staying safe

One of the central premises of the Children Act 2004 and the Every Child Matters (ECM) agenda is that a holistic approach needs to be achieved through multi-agency work to meet the needs of vulnerable young people (DfES 2004a). All local authorities are working towards enabling all young people in their jurisdiction to achieve the five ECM outcomes: being healthy; staying safe; enjoying and achieving; making a positive contribution; and achieving economic wellbeing.

Each outcome is relevant to sexually exploited young people, although because of their vulnerability, there has been a specific focus on 'staying safe' in this area of work. Section 3.5 of The 'Staying safe action plan' (DCSF 2008g) notes a parent's concern for the safety of their child, asking the government to focus on problems related to 'alcohol, sexual exploitation and drugs' (DCSF 2008g: 46). Sexual exploitation is identified as a 'new area' where services should be in place to respond quickly and effectively, noting that it is important that professionals 'know what signs to look for and where to go for more specialist information' (DCSF 2008g: 48). The action plan identifies a number of tasks for addressing sexual exploitation. It commits the government to implementing the prostitution strategy (HO 2006b), the cross-government 'Sexual violence and abuse action plan' (HMSO 2007) and to developing national service guidance on therapeutic and preventative interventions. It also commits to developing a guide for the Sexual Assault Referral Centers (SACRs) on providing services for children. Importantly, it commits to issuing the updated, rewritten SCIP guidance (DCSF 2009).

If followed through, these commitments could have great significance to sexually exploited young people, both in terms of developing and supporting therapeutic services to meet their mental health needs (see Chapter 8 for more detail on this) and for coordinating responses from police, health and child protection workers. However, they will remain as commitments on paper and fail to be integrated into a strategy for safeguarding sexually exploited young people if their implementation is not integrated into the heart of other policy developments that impact on service delivery to young people.

I refer to some of the developments within health, education and housing policy that have taken place in recent years to illustrate this point.

Safeguarding the health of sexually exploited children and young people

Research has identified a range of health problems experienced by sexually exploited children and young people. The work has noted that few will attend appointments with health clinics or sexual health clinics without dedicated key worker support. Even after sustained contact with a worker, many of the young people will fail to make or keep an appointment. Their lives can be too chaotic, they can be too angry or the exploitation that they are involved with might be so entrenched that they are prevented from attending (Scott and Skidmore 2006, Coy 2007).

The Department of Health has been active in developing a number of initiatives aimed at victims of violence to protect them from health problems caused by violence and, in particular, from sexual abuse. This includes working to improve contact with health professionals in extended schools, improving work under the specialist provision under the 'healthy schools' agenda, making health centres more 'child and young person' friendly and concentrating on the development of sexual health services for young people (Coleman and Brooks 2009). However, few of these initiatives will be meaningful to many sexually exploited children and young people unless they are supported by an outreach and support strategy that links health workers with the specialist sexual exploitation projects in the locality.

I develop this point below by looking at the potential benefits that could be gained by incorporating Child and Adolescent Mental Health Services (CAMHS) services with those targeted towards sexually exploited young people.

CAMHS services and work with sexually exploited children and young people

The recent review of CAMHS work (DCSF 2008a) noted that:

> for some groups the specialist knowledge related to the circumstances of their vulnerability maybe more easily accessed within a service dedicated to their particular group
>
> (DCSF 2008a: 74)

This notes the need for health workers to access knowledge about vulnerable young people. By default, this also suggests that it would be easier to access the young people at specialist youth service providers, rather than expecting them to make and keep appointments at generic universal health providers.

The review noted that children who face three or more stressful life events, such as family bereavement, divorce or family illness are three times more likely than other children to develop emotional and behavioural disorders; that children who lived in rented accommodation were more likely to have a persistent emotional disorder than those who did not; and that nearly 50% of children in local authority care have a clinically diagnosable mental health disorder, increasing to nearly 70% for those in residential care (DCSF 2008a: 20–21). These young people might be the very ones who have specific mental health needs and who might be less able to access and use generic health service provisions.

The review rightly points out that these data are associated with the social conditions identified, not caused by them. This is an important distinction as not all children and young people in rented accommodation or in care have mental health problems. The point is that the stresses associated with changing care/parenting contexts and with temporary or insecure accommodation can contribute to some young people being particularly vulnerable to mental health problems.

There is an increasing body of research identifying a wide range of diagnosed and undiagnosed mental health problems amongst sexually exploited children and young people, including self-harming behaviour, post-traumatic stress disorder, depression and suicidal feelings (Melrose and Barrett 2004, Chase and Statham 2006, Harper and Scott 2005, Scott and Skidmore 2006). Of 55 sexually exploited young women studied, 34 were regularly self-harming, 22 had been raped, all had problem alcohol use, 30 were regular heroin users and 18 had attempted suicide. They had a disproportionately large number of stress factors to try to manage, certainly over the three identified above as contributing to the development of mental health problems. Ten were managing between four and nine problems at any one time, 26 were managing between 10 and 13 problems, 17 managing 14 to 17 and 2 managing 18 to 21 problems (Pearce et al 2002: 23).

The problems facing the young people included missing from school and home, a history of familial sexual and/or physical abuse, disrupted parenting, experience of local authority care, chronic alcohol and drug problems. These findings are echoed in other research into the mental health needs of sexually exploited young people, including work with young men that identifies similar findings (Skidmore and Lillywhite 2006; and see Chapter 7).

Integrated CAMHS services

The 2008 review of CAMHS services notes that specialist and targeted interventions working at tiers three and four are directed towards young people with 'complex, severe and/or persistent needs' (DCSF 2008a: 18). These, I argue, need tailoring to address the needs of sexually exploited young people, accessing the young people in environments that are familiar to them and delivering the mental health service through sustained partnership/co-working arrangements with the staff of the dedicated project. This will mean cooperation with the key worker who has an already established relationship with the young people concerned.

For example, many case study reviews (Pearce et al 2002, Scott and Skidmore 2006) have noted that intensive support is needed to ensure that a young person attend to a mental health problem. The young person may deny the existence of a problem, thinking, for example, that cutting themselves is a helpful way to manage difficult thoughts and feelings. Then, if the young person does agree that there is a problem they may be so chaotic, confused or resistant to treatment that they forget, avoid or jeopardise the appointment. It is not uncommon for the young person to need constant reminding, support with transport, help in meeting and talking to the health care worker, support with after care, use of medication, follow-up treatment activities and with sustaining the necessary relationships with healthcare workers.

If the cross-government national plan (DH/HO 2001) was to be rewritten, it would consider how CAMHS services could support work being undertaken by other government departments, particularly the DCSF. This means ensuring that CAMHS are present on LSCBs subcommittees, are linking to the specialist dedicated services and are included in protocols directed to safeguarding these young people. It also means any national or local review of CAMHS services addressing how tiers three and four services are being used by sexually exploited children and young people.

Essentially, this requires a shift in the conceptual framework underpinning work with children and young people who experience a number of stresses in their lives. It means seeing these young people as in need of intensive support to treat mental health problems that may have been undiagnosed for a long period of time. This needs to run alongside child protection procedures, not operating in isolation from them. Safeguarding sexually exploited children and young people is a child protection issue but our conceptual framework needs to recognise that child protection cannot do it alone!

This does not mean pathologising the young people, it means identifying and addressing the severity of the range of problems they face. So for example, a young person in a sexually exploitative relationship may have an attachment disorder. This might be associated with experiences of disrupted parenting, previous abuse and addictive behaviours, and be aggravated by a number of foster care placement breakdowns. If this child is placed in a residential care home where there is a high turnover of poorly trained staff, the problems with attachment will not be addressed. This does not mean that residential care is not appropriate, but that the care home needs to provide staff trained in therapeutic work, supported by good and consistent supervision and resourced appropriately to manage highly complex case loads.

The level of care required within a care plan should reflect the level of distress experienced, recognising that the mental health needs require mental health interventions. Until we have a conceptual framework that recognises and addresses the range of sexually exploited, damaged and displaced young people's mental health needs, they will remain entrenched in damaging contexts that aggravate their problems.

Violence and healthcare initiatives

Other key initiatives taking place within the Department of Health also need to become more aware of the needs of sexually exploited young people. The department's aim to protect vulnerable victims, outlined in the Victims of Violence and Abuse Prevention Programme (DH 2008, Itzin 2008) note the need for services to be targeted towards vulnerable and abused young people. To be effective, this requires local service providers to engage with *how* this will happen: what it means to shift the approach from one relying on appointment led centre-based work to one that is flexible, engaged with drop in and outreach services and developed in partnership with dedicated services in touch with sexually exploited young people.

Similarly, initiatives relating to substance misuse prevention and treatment need specific targeted provision to support sexually exploited children and young people who have developing and entrenched problems with addiction. As noted, a high proportion of sexually exploited young people experience problem alcohol and drug use. Indeed, research has shown that abusers can actively encourage young people to become dependent upon drugs and alcohol, using the dependency as a mechanism for control (Melrose and Barrett 2004).

The aim to minimise problem substance misuse amongst children and young people is clearly stated within the ten-year drug strategy (2008–2018) where the four strands of work:

- Protecting communities through drug supply.
- Preventing harm to children and families affected by drug misuse.
- Delivering new approaches to drug treatment and social reintegration.
- Enhancing public information and community engagement.

should be fully integrated into preventative and direct intervention work with sexually exploited children and young people (HO 2008b). For a local drug action team to develop its strategy for work with young people without being fully integrated into the subcommittee for sexually exploited children young people, is a missed opportunity to prevent the escalation of both substance misuse and exploitation amongst these young people. It also misses the opportunity of building local knowledge networks about the location, distribution and purchase of illegal drugs within local communities. As noted in Chapter 7, young people themselves are one of the best sources of information about local networks sustaining informal economies (Pitts 2008).

The relationship between safety and health needs is an important component within the development of work to protect sexually exploited children and young people. However, as argued above, a sexually exploited child or young person will have other needs alongside health and safety. Engaging with child protection procedures to safeguard the individual from abuse is just one part of the strategy. Other strands mean engaging with them to look at their transition into independent living through supported access to training, employment and housing. These are equally important components to enabling children and young people to move away from exploitative situations.

Supported accommodation

Studies of sexually exploited children and young people show that access to safe, supported and permanent accommodation is central to their continued desistence from sexual exploitation. Of 55 sexually exploited young women, 18 were homeless (Pearce et al 2002). In most studies, many more than half the number of young people who are sexually exploited have histories of going missing, running from home and experiencing times without permanent secure accommodation (Chase and Statham 2005, Lebock and King 2006, Scott and Skidmore 2006).

The statistics of young people running from unsatisfactory homes, of needing respite accommodation and wanting to establish their independence while addressing their drug, alcohol or relationship problems are well researched. The Sheffield Safeguarding Children Board sexual exploitation service annual report 2006–2007 noted that one of the major indicators of risk of sexual exploitation is going missing from home or from care. Reported cases of missing from Sheffield between 2006 and 2007 were of two young people going missing between 10 and 15 times, 7 between 5 and 10 times and 21 between 1 and 5 times (Sheffield Safeguarding Children Board 2007).

Going missing

The annual report noted that the numbers would be an under-representation as many of the missing cases were not reported. For example, the Barnardos evaluation of its services, which also identified missing and homelessness as a key risk indicator for sexual exploitation, noted that many cases go unreported. They drew on a case of a young man who ran from home to escape his mother's aggression:

> she's been very violent towards him in the past, when she was drinking, that led him to go missing. He went missing from a young age, but just running you know, running out of the house just to get away. Mum didn't report him.
>
> (Scott and Skidmore 2006: 23)

The Barnardos evaluation of services notes that:

> going missing is the most immediate indicator of vulnerability to sexual exploitation. In the lives of many of the young people featured in this evaluation it indicated a crucial transition period during which they moved back and forth 'between worlds'
>
> (Scott and Skidmore 2006: 23)

If the focus is only on returning them to the abusive environment, they will continue to run and to place themselves in difficult, potentially exploitative situations. Following a full assessment, it might be better in some situations, to support the young person into making a transition from home to supported independent living. This means the safeguarding board working with housing services to address the needs of the minority of young people for whom home or foster care is no longer viable.

Worryingly, it is not uncommon for young people being looked after by the local authority to be temporarily placed in bed and breakfast accommodation, often placed in areas where the operation of informal economies around drug and sex markets are prevalent. Melrose and Barrett (2004) note studies of sexually exploited young people who were without safe accommodation, running from their family or care home and swapping sex for a bed for a night.

Homelessness and inadequate housing provision

The homelessness strategy outlined in 'Sustainable communities: settled homes, changing lives' (DCLG 2005) advocated the government's commitment to reducing homelessness amongst young people. It recognised that young people became homeless for a number of reasons and identified the need to prevent vulnerable young people from becoming homeless. This was updated in 2007 to ensure that use of bed and breakfast accommodation for 16 to 18 year olds was strongly discouraged, and that supported lodging schemes were used (DCLG 2007b).

Sometimes running from home is the result of abuse, sometimes it is the result of the pressures of overcrowding. More than one million children in Britain live in overcrowded, temporary, run down, damp or dangerous housing (Rice 2006). Eighty-one million homes in England fail to meet the government's decent home standard (DCLG 2007a) and more than 112,000 homeless children are living in temporary accommodation (DCLG 2008). Poor housing conditions are known to increase the risk of severe ill health and problems at school (Mitchell 2004, Harker 2006). Two-thirds of respondents to a Shelter survey among homeless households living in temporary accommodation said that their children had problems at school (Shelter 2008). However, despite these problems, Shelter is concerned that housing does not feature strongly enough with the ECM agenda and believes that:

> access to decent affordable housing must be at the heart of any strategy for improving the life chances of children and young people and reducing child poverty.
>
> (Shelter 2008: 3)

The Foyer movement

There are some examples where local authorities are developing partnership with housing providers to secure supported provision for the most vulnerable young people. For example, the foyer movement is beginning to work well with some local authorities and housing associations to provide supported independent living programmes for young people (www.foyer.net).The Swan Housing Group runs foyers for young people aged 16 to 25 years, which aim to help vulnerable young homeless people to gain confidence. A network of services provide 'back-up' provisions to the foyers, encouraging the young people to access education and employment possibilities while simultaneously supporting them to use their key worker in a way that builds positive relationships (Swan Housing Group 2007).

Supported foster care provision

Similarly, some local authorities are trying to develop trained and supported foster care provision, providing regular and sustained contact with the foster carer providing the home for the young person. As noted above, the conceptual shift that needs to take place here is from one that assumes that the young people have basic needs to one that recognises that the potential foster careers will be working with extremely disturbed and damaged young people. This is not labelling the young person as inadequate, but is recognising the intensive workload needed to manage the young person's behaviour. It is totally unrealistic to expect an untrained and unsupported foster carer to support the young person on their own.

Rutter et al note a randomised control trial of a specialised fostering programme in the USA which offered two-hour support sessions per week for foster carers of severely emotionally damaged young people. In addition, carers were given three to five hours of face-to-face contact and frequent phone conversations with support staff each week. Therapy was available for the family and/or the child and a significantly enhanced financial allowance was available to the foster carer. The young people improved their relationships with care providers, had reduced mental health problems and, although the intervention was expensive, it was noted that it resulted in a $10,000 reduction in hospitalisation costs per child (Rutter and Taylor 2002: 368). This trial gives an insight into the high levels of support and training needed to create positive outcomes for the foster carer and the young person concerned.

Some local authorities have long histories of developing good specialist foster care schemes, although many are directed at the younger age group. Manchester Link, for example, provides excellent therapeutic foster care for emotionally damaged young people but targets work with those under 14 years. Other foster and adoption agencies and associations provide specialist foster care, but unless these are directly linked into the local authority child sexual exploitation strategy and supported by dedicated outreach workers, they will be placing unrealistic pressures on the carers and the placement will run the risk of repeat breakdown.

One of the central themes identified by this work to date is that the essential component to both specialist foster care and independent living schemes is that they are supported by named dedicated staff. These staff must understand the dynamics facing the young person and be in a position to provide on going support work with the young person and a 'crisis intervention' rapid response to cover specific problems as they arise.

Education and training

Sex and relationship education will be made compulsory for all secondary schools, preventative education having progressed to include a special briefing on preventing sexual exploitation (Lewis and Martinez 2006). Early identification of young people at risk of exploitation can help to ensure that referrals are made to safeguarding boards and that interventions follow to divert the young person from harm (Scott and Skidmore 2006). The work of the Barnardos project 'Sexually Exploited Children Outreach Services' (SECOS) shows that once local education staff are trained to recognise the early warning signs, the sexual exploitation indicators, referrals to the dedicated project for preventative work increase (SECOS 2008).

While schools have a role to play in early identification, their response to young people who are truanting or going missing is equally important. Research argues that being out of school and employment makes the young people particularly vulnerable to sexual exploitation. Those who are known to be exploited are also known to have a history of truanting from school or of being excluded from school (Leboch and King 2006). Significant developments have been made through the DCSF to try to address the needs of 14 to 18 year olds in their transition from school to work, placing particular focus on the needs of vulnerable young people (DSCF 2008e, Rathbone 2008). Placing particular focus on the needs of children and young people who are not in education, employment or training (NEET), the government figures suggest that the number of NEETs have fallen from 10.4% to 9.4% in 2007 (DCSF 2008c: 2). However, overall the numbers of NEETS have increased, with those who had persistent absenteeism from school being seven times more likely to be NEET (DCSF 2008c: 3). In 2006–2007, there were 1,043,000 young adults (under 25 years) of NEET status, an increase of 131,000 since 1997 (Field and White 2007: 20). The number of young people currently classified as NEET but who are not claiming Job Seeker Allowance or taking part in a New Deal programme are also rising (Field and White 2007: 21). Moreover, there are concerns that the implementation of the strategy might be problematic as it requires dedicated resources at a local level (Yates and Payne 2007).

The developing NEET strategy is being structured around four themes: a) careful tracking to identify those at risk; b) personalised guidance and support; c) enabling the young people to access suitable provision; and d) tackling barriers to learning. It notes the need to provide more targeted and intensive support for those young people with particular barriers to 'participation or re-engagement' (DCSF 2008c: 3). For this to realistically impact on sexually exploited young people, these targeted and intensive support strategies need to be linked into the protocol for safeguarding sexually exploited young people in a meaningful way. That is, once a young person who is off the school role and out of employment is identified, education and employment workers need to be available to link with the dedicated specialist project for sexually exploited young people in the area, accompanying staff on outreach and drop-in sessions and be able to develop sustained relationships with the young people to build trust, confidence, raise self-esteem and explain the value of training and employment.

In much of the above debate I have referred to policy initiatives being possible if linked to dedicated services where workers are trained and employed to support sexually exploited children and young people. However, as noted, most local authorities do not have access to such a service (Jago and Pearce 2008). The policy initiatives themselves are worthless if they cannot be put into action and resourced to achieve their laudable aims. These policy developments mentioned above in health, housing, education and employment are just a small section of the many initiatives developed since 2000 to improve the protection of children and young people from abuse, to improve access of NEETS to mainstream services, to improve the mental, physical and sexual health of the young people concerned and to address the longer-term housing and independent living needs of young people in line with the five outcomes specified within the ECM agenda (DfES 2004a). What is needed now is a conceptual shift that encourages accommodation of the needs of sexually exploited children and young people within each of the five outcomes, not only the more obvious one of 'staying safe'. For local authorities to achieve this, there needs to be a 'model of good practice' demonstrated by central government.

Central government model of multi-agency work

One way for safeguarding boards to be supported in developing multi-agency work would be for central government to 'model' a joined up approach. This would mean that there was a cross-government strategy to protect children and young people from sexual exploitation, as initiated in the 2001 national plan. Distressingly, this has been abandoned, leaving the various strategies (a selection of which are outlined above) developing through separate departments, often repeating the same aims through different and separated strands of work, failing to create a joined up approach at a central, yet alone a local level.

Although the redrafted SCIP guidance, 'Safeguarding children and young people from sexual exploitation' (DCSF 2009) is one step towards this, it is focused on the work from one of the many government departments and is working to the safeguarding agenda rather than providing a forum for sustained joined up work between all departments.

The reason that this is important is that while work with prevention and intervention with sexually exploited children is seen predominantly as a child protection issue, interventions that can offer support on housing and accommodation, on training and employment, on emotional and physical wellbeing will, at worst, be missed or at best, be delivered as disjointed and uncoordinated. Unfortunately, the current dominant focus on 'grooming' for sexual exploitation can inadvertently encourage exploitation to be seen *only* as an issue of abuse (therefore one of child protection), rather than encouraging a holistic perspective to address the young person's associated needs.

As noted in Chapter 1, there are other 'routes into' exploitation, including responding to push factors such as attempting to escape from poverty, or pull factors, such as asserting a perceived (although invariably misguided) agency in achieving independence and freedom through sexual activity. This does not mean that the young person is no less damaged in the process, but does mean that interventions need more expertise and resources than just those provided under the umbrella of child protection. While the traditional child protection agencies might be somewhat equipped to respond to the younger vulnerable victim who is groomed into exploitation, they may be less equipped to work with the challenging teenager who wants to run from home and decide for themselves how, when and under what circumstances they swap or sell sex. For the range of sexually exploited children and young people to achieve the five ECM outcomes, education, training and employment services, housing services and health services need to join together to ensure a holistic approach to support.

'New' technologies

The other major change that has occurred since the SCIP guidance of 2000 is the range of methods that can be used to access young people for sexual exploitation. As the use of 'new' technologies such as the mobile phone and the internet has grown, there have been other ways for abusive adults to contact and groom young people into exploitation. This has led to a recognition, identified within the definition of sexual exploitation given by the National Working Group for Sexually Exploited Children Young People (NWG 2008) and used in the DCSF guidance (2009). The new definition recognises that:

> Child Sexual exploitation can occur through use of technology without the child's immediate recognition; for example the persuasion to post sexual images on the internet/mobile phones with no immediate payment or gain.
>
> (NWG 2008)

The threat of technology?

Although we have limited research into the use of the internet for the purpose of sexual exploitation, we have increasing awareness of the vulnerability of some young people to sexual exploitation through use of 'new technologies' (Palmer and Stacey 2004). They noted the dangers facing many young people, particularly boys and young men, who were vulnerable to exploitation on the internet. Chase and Statham (2005) note a study by O'Connell (2003) of young people's use of chat rooms over a five-year period. O'Connell developed the use of the term 'cybersexploitation' to cover the grooming of children in cyberspace, noting that cyberspace creates larger social networks where there are fewer controls for protecting vulnerable children.

Concern for the welfare of young people using social networking sites (SNSs) has proliferated. In the USA, the house of representatives voted by an overwhelming majority to ban, with few exceptions, the use of SNSs in schools, libraries and other publicly funded resources. However, this may only force young people to use SNSs in places where they cannot be supervised. Responding to the concern of abuse over the internet, safety awareness programmes have been developed to encourage young people to be mindful of the dangers that they may face and to educate parents and carers about how to best protect their children (Bryon 2008). Bryon is careful to consider whether the concern of potential exploitation can create an unnecessary culture of fear and, if poorly handled, can divide adult and adolescent age groups from each other (Bryon 2008).

The important consideration is that due caution of the risks involved may not reach those young people who are the most vulnerable to sexual exploitation. Associated to this is the concern that the processes for recording harm and potential abuse are not fully incorporated into safeguarding children boards' procedures. This has resulted in a DCSF publication targeted at local safeguarding boards in an effort to improve the protection of the most vulnerable (DCSF 2008d).

The police have also responded to the concern that the online environment can be harmful to vulnerable young people. The Child Exploitation Online Protection agency (CEOP) was created in 2006 to coordinate 'law enforcement's response to child sex abuse' (CEOP 2006: 6). It is closely linked to other police units such as the serious sex offenders unit, the paedophile online investigation team and with the serious organised crime agency (SOCA). Whilst much of its work focuses on protection from harm 'online' it also recognises that there is a false distinction between on- and offline abuse.

CEOP has a brief to develop education, awareness raising and victims' support as well as bringing offenders to account; to identify, locate and protect children and young people from sexual exploitation and online abuse; to engage and empower young people's parents and the community through information and education; to protect children and young people through the provisions of specialist information and support to professionals, families, industry and the community; to enforce the law by bringing offenders to justice and acting to disrupt and deter future offending; and to enhance existing responses to the sexual exploitation and online abuse of children and young people by developing a safer online environment by design, and the better management of offenders (CEOP 2006: 7).

That these broad aims exist is commendable. For them to be effective at a local level there needs to be communication between local police officers, dedicated sexual exploitation workers and child protection workers.

Conclusion

In this chapter I have argued that although progress has been made in our knowledge and understanding of sexual exploitation since 2000, we still fall short of providing an integrated service across the country. Many localities fail to identify the need for a dedicated service for the young people and continue to miss the early warning signs of sexual exploitation as demonstrated by some young people in school, health clinics and youth service provisions. Also, although there are some examples of child protection services and police working well together, sharing intelligence and disrupting and prosecuting abusers, they are in the minority and are often short lived, depending upon the commitment and dedication of a small number of staff (Jago and Pearce 2008). Although it is helpful, if not essential, for child sexual exploitation to be seen as a concern for child protection practitioners, this is only half the story.

Two conceptual shifts need to take place. One needs to shift awareness to the severity of the mental health needs of the young people. This would mean that interventions recognise the frailty of the existence of many of the young people, ensuring that staff who are working with them are appropriately trained and supported. It would mean recognising the damage that can be done by placing vulnerable young people in inappropriate accommodation, such as bed and breakfast accommodation and some residential care settings. Again, to clarify, this is not to say that all residential care placements are problematic, but that many are known to have a high turnover of staff and to be locations targeted by abusers.

The second conceptual shift to be made is to recognise the range of needs of the sexually exploited young person. As well as being victims of abuse, the young people have potential to be active agents of their own destiny. With support and good, child-centred health, education and employment services, they are capable of building on their own resources. For this to take place, child protection, health, education, employment, housing and police services need to work together.

Central government can play a major role in supporting this to happen by creating an up-to-date national plan for safeguarding children and young people from sexual exploitation that both models 'joined up' work and provides a context for implementation and review of cross-department initiatives.

As noted, one of the areas that is under development is the impact of the relationship between experiences of violence and general wellbeing. I turn to look at how young people's experience of violence in relationships has been understood in chapter four. Before doing this, I explore one further 'new' development – the trafficking of children and young people for sexual exploitation.

3   The trafficking of children and young people: Implications for work with sexually exploited children and young people

Freedom

I'm as free as a bird
But one year ago
I was like a bird in a cage
Screaming 'let me out
I want to be free from this life'.
But I thought I was trapped
But all I had to do was sing
And people would start noticing me
And then someone noticed me and let me
Out of my cage.
Now I'm as free as a bird
And I'm not trapped in that life anymore
You can do it as well
It's true you know.
     (Denise, aged 17, Street Matters 2000)

Introduction

Concerns about 'new' and different processes through which young men and women can be sexually exploited, have attracted increasing attention in the last decade. As noted above, the exploitation and the trafficking of young people for work in prostitution has a long history. However, a renewed focus has been placed on the vulnerability of young people who are trafficked into and within the UK resulting in a sudden plethora of publications and policy guidance documents (HO 2006b, Harris and Robinson 2007, CEOP et al 2007, ECPAT 2007, Craig 2008, DCSF 2008e).

This chapter will focus on the question of safeguarding children and young people who are trafficked into the country, referring in particular to those who are trafficked for the purpose of sexual exploitation. I want to identify some of the tensions that exist within debates about trafficked young people: tensions about the identification, referral and resource allocation to meet young people's short and long-term needs. Central to these tensions are questions of risk, victimhood and young people's agency. For example,

- Is the young person who is trafficked into the UK 'kidnapped' from abroad as a victim of 'modern-day slavery', or are they, possibly with their family, taking some dangerous, ill-informed risks by paying traffickers to take them away from poverty and war?
- Is a UK national young person (holding British citizenship) visiting an older exploitative adult (whom they might refer to as a boyfriend or girlfriend) in another UK city, a victim of trafficking for the purpose of sexual exploitation? Or are they someone who sees themselves as looking for an adventure, seeking somewhere better than home to stay, exploring for love, comfort or financial reward?

As argued in Chapters 1 and 2, these questions do not undermine the need for sexual exploitation to be understood as sexual abuse. The implications for child protection need to be addressed by safeguarding boards. Neither do they negate the responsibility to protect children and young people from harm. Rather, they encourage a young person-centered approach to policy and practice that is sensitive to the specific developmental stages of adolescence, asking how the young person sees and understands the situation that they are in.

I raise these questions not to challenge the view that the young person is a victim of abuse from adults who are committing offences, but rather to ask how the young person themselves might understand the processes involved. It is important to raise these questions as I have a concern that the needs of trafficked young people might be misconstrued in discourses of 'slavery'.

This chapter looks at the formal definitions of a trafficked young person; some of the research and policy initiatives that have been developed to guide practice in the field; and at research that has taken place in the UK to help develop an understanding of the issues facing the young people concerned.

Definitions of trafficked young people: The UN context

Children's and young people's right to freedom from being abducted, forcibly moved and exploited was clearly spelt out in the 1989 UN convention on the rights of the child. Identifying a child as anyone under the age of 18 years, the convention extended civil, cultural, economic, political and social rights to children (UN 1989). The convention sets out these rights in 54 articles and two optional protocols. Articles 34, 35 and 36 give young people under 18 years the right to be free from sexual abuse, from exploitation and from being kidnapped or sold, providing the backdrop to the developing discourse of 'trafficking' into and within the UK for the purpose of sexual exploitation. A child-friendly description of each article is available for young people to access and use (www.rcmp-grc.gc.ca/pdfs/NCD-poster_e.pdf and www.unicef.org.uk). This international framework has been important in providing leadership on the need to protect young people from being trafficked.

The convention has been ratified by 191 out of 193 countries, territories and states, although not all without some reservations on specific articles. The UK signed in 1991, although with a controversial immigration reservation on Article 22 which guaranteed protection for young refugees. The government reviewed this reservation in line with changes in child care and immigration legislation (The Children Act 2004; The UK Borders Act 2007). Section 21 of the UK Borders Act 2007 called for a code of practice issued that is designed to ensure that the then Border and Immigration Agency (BIA) (now UK Border Agency) takes appropriate steps to ensure that while children are in the UK they are safe from harm. There was criticism levelled at the tardy response to lifting the reservation to Article 22, with pressure building on the government to ensure that children and young people are safe from harm at the point of entry to the UK (ECPAT 2008).

In February 2008, the Council of Europe (COE) convention against human trafficking came into force. It was written as treaties series 197 in 2005 with the aim of promoting international cooperation on action against trafficking, to prevent and combat the trafficking in human beings and to protect the human rights of victims of trafficking. In December 2008 the UK government became the 20th state to ratify the convention, with it enacted in April 2009. The COE Convention Against Human Trafficking is being implemented with an accompanying new national referral mechanism (NRM) to help staff identify cases of trafficking.

A further United Nations Protocol titled the 'UN convention on Transnational Organised Crime' was published in 2000. This clarified the need to prevent, suppress and punish trafficking in persons. It advances a three-pronged approach: preventing trafficking in human beings, prosecuting offenders, and supporting victims. The Palermo Protocol of 2003 supplemented the 2000 convention, Article 3 defining the trafficking of people as the 'Recruitment, transportation, transfer, harbouring or receipt of persons by means of threat, use of force, coercion, abduction, fraud, deception, abuse of power for the purpose of exploitation'. It notes in Article 3a that:

> Exploitation shall include, at a minimum, the exploitation of the prostitution of others or other forms of sexual exploitation, forced labour or services, slavery or practices similar to slavery, servitude or the removal of organs.
>
> (Article 3a, UN 2003)

Recognising the impact of abuse and violence, the agreement clarifies that if the conditions outlined in Article 3a have been applied, the consent of the victim is irrelevant. It also notes that:

> The recruitment, transportation, transfer, harbouring or receipt of a child for the purpose of exploitation shall be considered 'trafficking in human beings' even if this does not involve any of the means set forth in subparagraph (a) of this article
>
> (Palermo Protocol Article 3c, UN 2003)

This Palermo Protocol has been used as the established definition of the trafficking of young people. As noted in the Department of Children Schools and Families (DCSF) guidance on 'Safeguarding children who may have been trafficked' (DCSF 2008e), the Palermo Agreement:

> establishes children as a special case. Any child transported for exploitative reasons is considered to be a trafficking victim, whether or not that have been forced or deceived. This is partly because it is not considered possible for children to give informed consent. Even when a child understands what has happened, they may still appear to submit willingly to what they believe to be the will of their parents or accompanying adults. It is important that these children are protected also
>
> (DCSF 2008e: 6)

Returning for a moment to the question of whether the young person can give informed consent, whether they can have some role in decision-making in the process (perhaps as an attempt to achieve the human right to live without poverty, war or violence), it is helpful to consider other situations where a young person is considered capable of giving informed consent. For example, the Fraser guidelines produced certain criteria by which a young person could give informed consent about their future. Specifically focused on the questions of contraception for under 16s, the debate about Gillick competency and the resulting Fraser guidelines raised the question about when and how young people's views should be accommodated in debates about their future (Wheeler 2006).

The issues involved in a young person giving informed consent to using contraceptives as opposed to giving informed consent to illegal trafficking are different. However, interventions that uncritically accept a 'victim approach' and that do not seek to hear whether, how and why the young person might have been trafficked, is to undermine the importance of seeking young people's opinion in making decisions about their future. It might be that the young person was deciding themselves that they wanted to take some risks to escape war and poverty and that in so doing, they saw themselves as taking some responsibility for their future.

Trafficking of children and young people: The UK context

A number of recent initiatives in the UK have helped to raise the profile of young people who have been trafficked into, within and out from the UK. The government launched both the Child Exploitation and Online Protection Centre (CEOP) and the UK Human Trafficking Centre (UKHTC) in 2006 as initiatives to protect children from online abuse and to prevent the trafficking of human beings. These centres were launched prior to the publication of the UK Human Trafficking Action Plan (HO and Scottish Government 2007c) which, now updated (HO and Scottish Government 2008), also has a specific chapter on the trafficking of children and young people.

CEOP works across the UK and maximises international links to combine police powers with expertise of business sectors, government, specialist charities and other interested organisations. Its focus is to challenge child sex abuse and to develop awareness of and better policing of organised abuse through use of the internet (www.ceop.gov.uk). It includes a concern to protect children and young people from sexual exploitation. As such, it invests interest in issues relating to the trafficking of young people. It produced an important 'scoping exercise' that gave an overview of the suspected scale of the problem of the trafficking of children and young people both into and within the UK (CEOP et al 2007).

The UKHTC was established specifically to focus on the prevention and prosecution issues relating to the trafficking of human beings. It was, in part, a response to the impact of the police operation Pentameter One which involved 55 police forces working together over a three-month period. Working with a coordinated police response across the country it identified 84 trafficked women, including 12 children between 14 and 17 years. Two hundred and thirty-two arrests were made. The operation revealed concern about the UK being a through and destination country for human trafficking and is being repeated in Pentameter 2. The focus of Pentameter 2 is on trafficking for the purpose of sexual exploitation but also carries a strategic aim of increasing knowledge and understanding of all forms of trafficking. The UKHTC provides a central point for operational coordination in relation to the trafficking in human beings.

The UKHTC has recently developed a specific working group to focus on the internal trafficking of young people within the UK for the purpose of sexual exploitation (www.ukhtc.org). While the 'internal trafficking' of young people is important to address, there are distinctions that need to be maintained between the needs of indigenous UK nationals trafficked for the purpose of sexual exploitation and the needs of children from abroad. I suggest that there are two distinct forms of internal trafficking of young people in the UK. These involve addressing the somewhat different needs and issues of young people who are:

- *Trafficked from abroad.* These young people may not speak English, may have little knowledge of the UK support systems available through Children's Services, may have come from 'home' cultures (and climates) that are profoundly different to those in the UK and may have experienced violence and abuse during their journey. They are unlikely to have any knowledge of a local peer group or family/care network that they could have any access to within the UK. They will be moved on within the UK after arrival and therefore defined as 'internally trafficked'.
- *Indigenous UK nationals trafficked within the UK.* The focus has, in the main, been on UK nationals trafficked for the purpose of sexual exploitation (as according to the Sexual Offences Act 2003). However, further work needs to be carried out to identify the potential scale of the trafficking of UK nationals for other forms of exploitation. Most of these young people will be English speaking (as a second if not first language). They will, in the

main, have a knowledge or familiarity with different cultures in the UK and will have some awareness of a local peer group, family or care network within the UK.

When using the concept of 'internal trafficking' it is important that these distinctions are held in mind so that resources can be distributed to meet the needs of the different young people concerned. This reflects similar concerns within studies of migration which are invariably split into two different bodies of work – that of international migration between countries and internal migration within countries (King et al 2008). A review of the literature suggested that there were inherent difficulties in trying to apply one single theory of migration to explain all forms of migration across the globe.

Work emerging from these initiatives has raised awareness of the need to both protect children from abroad and UK nationals from trafficking. The NSPCC Child Trafficking Advice and Information Help Line (see NSPCC for further information); the DCSF publication of guidance for LSCBs on safeguarding children who may have been trafficked (DCSF 2008e); and findings from recent research projects (ECPAT UK 2007, CEOP 2007, Harris and Robinson 2007, Pearce et al 2009) have all contributed to raising the need for improved law enforcement interventions that can disrupt and prosecute traffickers. I draw below on some of the key findings that have come from this body of work, focusing on issues relating to the trafficking of young people for sexual exploitation.

Protecting trafficked children and young people for sexual exploitation

Although it is clear that young people are trafficked for reasons such as domestic servitude, benefit fraud and labour exploitation, the focus here is on sexual exploitation. A range of legislation is available to protect children and young people from harm through sexual exploitation and trafficking.

For example, Sections 57 to 59 of the Sexual Offences Act 2003 identify it an offence to intentionally arrange or facilitate movement of a person for the purpose of sexual exploitation. The Violent Crime Reduction Act 2006 introduced the power of forfeiture and detention of vehicles, ships and aircraft used in trafficking for sexual exploitation. Although, as noted above, there have been tensions around the UK compliance with the UN convention of the rights of the child, the recent code of good practice issued by the UK Border Agency means that trafficked children and young people should receive immediate referral to children's services for protection (UKBA 2007).

As well as the UK Action Plan on Tackling Human Trafficking having consideration of the needs of young people who are trafficked into and within the UK, the UK Staying Safe Action Plan 2008 notes the need to improve the provision of a 'safety net' and of safe places for young people who go missing from home (DCSF 2008g: 45).

Importantly the action plan notes the need for new guidelines for missing young people to help raise awareness amongst all children's services (DCSF 2008g: 52). The DSCF publication on safeguarding children who may have been trafficked also sets out criteria for local authorities to follow, explaining the legislation available to support their practice. The guidance provides a range of flow charts to guide practitioners through the use of Sections 17, 20 and 47 of the Children Act 1989. Importantly, it sets out a framework for preventing the inappropriate use of private foster care arrangements.

Despite this helpful policy and legislative framework, research suggests that practitioners feel poorly equipped to identify and respond to the needs of young people who have been trafficked, and local authorities struggle to find funding streams to support appropriate initiatives that might be developed to provide the consistent and intense levels of care that are needed (Pearce et al 2009).

Slavery and the human rights agenda

Recent debate has increasingly conflated trafficking and slavery discourses. There is a potential worry about this. Such conflation can cause emotive responses to the problems that cloud or confuse the actual circumstances of some of the young people concerned. There is no doubt that some young people are trafficked into the country against their will, through use of force, violence and/or coercion. Others might find themselves to be exploited at the point of entry. Their passports, identity cards and other documents might be forcibly removed and they might be placed into exploitative, 'slave'-like situations.

As the exploitation of the young person is central to the definition of trafficking, it is inevitable that there are overlaps with 'slave'-like situations. Indeed, it is these conditions that separate the experiences of a trafficked child from one who has been smuggled, or who is an unaccompanied asylum-seeking child (UASC). The UK Action Plan on Tackling Human Trafficking has four main proposals: prevention, investigation, law enforcement, and prosecution (including 'internal trafficking') (HO and Scottish Government 2007 8–11). It says that the 'trafficking in human beings is an abhorrent crime' and that it is a form of 'modern-day slavery' (page 4). Noting that its publication date coincided with the 200th-year anniversary of the abolition of slavery in the British Empire the action plan intends to make the UK a hostile environment for any forms of human trafficking.

Similarly, reference to a range of websites of organisations working on protecting victims of trafficking shows a particular concern about the abuse of women and children through sex slavery (Stop the traffic, UKHTC), a concern often picked up by the media. The combinations of the words 'sex' and 'slave' are particularly emotive, attracting attention in the same way that pictures of girls in a short skirt standing by men's cars will do (see Chapter 7 for more detail).

However, a little caution is needed to prevent some of the situations faced by some of the young people from being taken out of context. If the young person or/and their family wanted to escape from war, extreme poverty and violence, they may have taken great risks in attempting to leave, expressing voices of resilience and anger about their previous conditions in their countries of origin. They may not understand themselves to be 'slaves' and may not want a 'rescue' attempt to underestimate their fear of return to war and violence.

So, at the heart of the trafficking of children and young people, debate is the right of the child to live a life free from poverty, violence and abuse (UN 1989). This can create a conflict for the young person as the desire to live without violence and poverty may draw them and their family into taking the risk of using traffickers. While some young people are 'kidnapped' or 'bought' against their will by organised criminal networks, the desire for access to this basic human right of living free from poverty, violence and abuse can drive some young people (perhaps encouraged by their family) to seek any method of movement away from home.

Indeed, the very notion of 'home' needs some deconstruction as the qualities associated with 'home' may not be applicable to young people trafficked into the country from abroad, or to indigenous UK nationals who are trafficked internally for sexual exploitation. This is explored by Breuil (2008: 229) in her work where she explores child-centered perspectives of trafficking.

> Trafficking children then, forcefully tearing them away from their imagined safe homes and placing them in an environment imagined as vile, danger-ous, (sexually) exploitative and evil, might not only or mainly outrage us because we are empathetic towards the child, but also because it invades our own social order (O'Connell-Davidson, 2005): it strikes at the roots of what we consider to be worthwhile in life and what we would like to pre-serve. However, this image of child trafficking is based on social construc-tions of how we see children and what we think is their proper place in the world. These are not necessarily untrue, but they are normative, and as such historically and culturally specific

The 'normative' image of home as a safe place cannot be assumed as true for all young people, particularly those whose 'homes' have been destroyed or attacked by violence and abuse.

Reasons for being trafficked

The United Nations Children's Fund (UNICEF) notes the relationships between poverty and discrimination and the forced movement and the sale of children and young people (UNICEF 2006). It encourages a holistic approach to the problem to address contributing factors that push young people into being trafficked such as underdevelopment, poverty, economic disparities, inequitable socioeconomic structure, dysfunctioning families, lack of education, urban–rural migration, gender discrimination and irresponsible adult sexual beha-viour. These are all noted as playing an important role in understanding and addressing the trafficking of persons (UNICEF 2005, 2006) and were endorsed in the 'Council of Europe Convention on Action against Trafficking in Human Beings' (COE May 2005), which stressed the need for a '"multidisciplinary co-ordination approach" between police, immigration, social services, courts, NGOs and others' (COE 2005: 42).

Rafferty (2007) helpfully identifies three main causes to the trafficking of persons, focusing specifically on the 'push factors': those factors that encourage a young person to consider taking risks to leave their current location. Focusing on child trafficking in South East Asia, she draws on UNICEF and Terre des Hommes work of 2006 to show child trafficking in South Eastern Europe to be linked with:

- Immediate causes (decisions made by children, adolescents, their parents and other individuals around them).
- Underlying causes (conditions that influence such decisions by individuals including unawareness of risks involved and trust in people from the same community).
- Structural causes (economic crisis, social exclusion, gender discrimination, weak legal and social protection systems)

(Rafferty 2007: 401)

Focusing on the impact of poverty, she identifies Dottridge's work of 2002 to describe how:

> endemic rural poverty in Africa often causes poor families to sell their children to traffickers, hoping for improved circumstances for their children
>
> (Rafferty 2007: 403)

She notes that according to the US Department of State 2007, India has the world's largest labour trafficking problems. She refers to Poudel and Carryer (2000) who argue that the trafficking of young Nepalese girls is not only con-nected to economic poverty but is rooted in regional gender politics and sexual inequalities (Rafferty 2007: 403).

It is important to be reminded of the 'push' factors: the reasons that young people and their families might be looking for escape from the country of origin, as well as the 'pull' factors: the demand for cheap or free labour, for recruits into petty crime, and for vulnerable children to exploit through sexual abuse (Anderson and O'Connell-Davidson 2003, O'Connell-Davidson 2005). As noted by Beddoe in her work for ECPAT UK on trafficked young people into the UK, the desire to come to the UK, or indeed to escape from poverty and war must not be seen as an illegal migration issue:

> It is global human rights abuse that requires national, regional and inter-national co-operation to protect children
>
> (ECPAT 2007: 8)

This work informs us of the impact that poverty and war can have on young people and their families who might take enormous risks to leave their place of origin, risks that might include collaborating with criminal traffickers. It helps us to understand some of the dynamics that face the young person who might feel unable to return to their country of origin, and whose relationship with organised or informal criminal networks may be linked with their families' desire for them to have a better life.

This does not collude with the unacceptable exploitation taking place for trafficked young people. More, it asks for a broader understanding of the context within which trafficking takes place and of how trafficking exists for a variety of push and pull reasons.

Countries of origin

Research has suggested that, in the main, trafficked children and young people are of African or Asian nationality, with some being from Eastern Europe and Jamacia (Dowling et al 2007: 11).

The CEOP scoping exercise that looked into the circumstances of 330 suspected cases of trafficking of children into the UK in 2007 noted that where information was forthcoming, it was evident that vulnerable children were reported to have come from broken families or destitute circumstances (CEOP et al 2007). CEOP noted a similar focus in its scoping exercise into trafficked young people. Data were found from 41 police forces and law enforcement agencies, 20 Children's Services, 21 Border and Immigration Agencies and eight non-governmental organisations (NGOs) in the UK. The research team gathered case data from these agencies of child trafficking that came to their attention between March 2005 and December 2006, and where the victim was still under the age of 18 years in March 2005. Qualitative data from these agencies were also sought and, in particular, from practitioners who have experience of working with child trafficking cases.

Recognising the problems with identifying trafficked young people and the time that it takes before a young person may say that they have been trafficked, the scoping exercise created four levels of probability of young people being trafficked. Of the 330 young people assessed:

- Seventy were placed in Level One: low probability – missing children referred by an agency as a possible case with no supporting evidence.
- Seventy were placed in Level Two: medium probability matching two or three indicators such as refusing to talk, being cared for by adults who are not parents when relationship is poor.
- Eighty-five were placed in Level Three: high probability – law enforcement investigations consistent with recognised child trafficking profiles.
- One hundred and five were placed in Level Four: very high probability – clear evidence of being trafficked.

Those who came from African countries, of whom Eastern African countries are highlighted as the third largest source region for the trafficking of children to the UK:

> reported having been orphaned, victims or prisoners of war, victims of sexual and physical abuse, forced into marriages, victimised by traumatic traditions such as female genital mutilation (FGM) and victims of police and social brutality most of the children came from
>
> (CEOP et al 2007: 22)

The study noted that the UK is a significant transit and destination country for trafficked children, noting the biggest source counties to be China, Western and Eastern Africa, Eastern Europe and Russia. Forty-four source countries in total were identified in the study and varied in regions, mainly consisting of the Far East, South East Asia, Central Asia, South Asia, West Africa, Eastern Europe and the Baltic states (CEOP et al 2007: 5). In total, 85% (276 children) were found to be between the ages of 15 and 17 years. Twenty-four children were found to be between 13 and 14 years of age, 14 were documented as 12 years and under, the youngest being a 9-month-old baby (CEOP et al 2007: 6).

ECPAT's work found similar patterns with the majority of the young people in their study of 80 suspected cases coming from Africa and East Asia (ECPAT 2007: 7). Thirty-eight of the 50 young people who were suspected of being trafficked in the West Sussex review were 16 or 17 years, 62% (21) were of Chinese origin, 12 were from Liberia and 7 were from India. Most presented as separated children, either as unaccompanied minors or with adults who were not holding parental responsibility for them (Harris and Robinson 2007).

A comprehensive report into the health needs of trafficked women identified a range of health and social care issues. Because of previous experiences of abuse and sexual and physical violence, many did not necessarily feel safe to return to their country of origin (Zimmerman et al 2006). Stressing the need for destination countries to provide sensitive healthcare provisions that could meet the level of trauma and abuse that the trafficked women had experienced, the report highlights the sexual and mental health needs of the women involved.

Two hundred and seven women were interviewed from 14 different source countries. Eighty-nine per cent of the women identified were trafficked from European states (9.2% of which were EU member states in 2006). Fifty three per cent were trafficked to European Union member states, 16% of whom were trafficked to the UK.

Adolescents between the ages of 15 and 17 years made up 12% of the total sample, and a further 21% were aged between 18 and 20 years. The following findings were made:

- Sixty per cent of the women noted that they had received violence in their country of origin prior to being trafficked (including 32% who had been sexually abused and 50% who had experienced physical assault).

- Just over one-quarter of the women (26%) reporting a forced or coerced sexual experience after the age of 15 years prior to being trafficked.

However, being trafficked was no relief from the violence and intimidation. Noting that the 'Loss of freedom is a defining feature of trafficking' (Zimmerman et al 2006: 11) noted that only 3% of the sample said that they were 'always free'.

As with the notion of 'home', they had conflicting understandings of the notion of freedom. For example, 'I could go out when I wanted to, but only with someone' (Zimmerman et al 2006: 11).

Highlighting the important need for EU countries to address the problem of trafficked people, and of improving health and social care responses to them, UNICEF published a study of eight countries' awareness of and responses to human trafficking (UNICEF 2005). Covering Albania, Bosnia and Herzegovina, Bulgaria, Croatia, the former Yugoslav Republic of Macedonia, Moldova, Romania and Serbia and Montenegro (including the UN-administered province of Kosovo) the study noted that the awareness of trafficking within these countries was limited.

It claimed that the awareness-raising activities that were taking place were ad hoc information campaigns run by different organisations who often did not have much contact with each other. While recognising the value of many campaigns, the report noted that few had been evaluated and lessons learnt had not been shared. It argued that effective reintegration programmes were rare and that despite help, most trafficking victims return home to poverty, discrimination, lack of education, few job prospects and, sometimes, political conflict and unrest. The findings showed that as law enforcement advanced, traffickers became more skilled, and victims less willing to seek assistance as they were fearful of repatriation, deportation and stigmatisation.

Gender and trafficked young people

It has been noted that 'research that has been published in the UK to date has tended to focus on the trafficking of women/children for sexual exploitation' (Dowling et al 2007: 1). Boys and young men have tended to be overlooked in safeguarding provisions because:

- The dominance of a radical feminist theoretical model that assumes trafficking to be 'gender related' violence (see O'Connell Davidson 2005 for further critique of the radical feminist position). This positions women as the victims of male violence, overshadowing the needs of young men who might be victims of such abuse.
- Entrenched stereotypes of gender-specific roles, crime and criminality mean that neither boys, nor practitioners, may expect young men to be victims of trafficking. They may not be equipped with a language or confidence to approach boys as victims of abuse (see Chapter 7 for further discussion of these issues) and, as a result, boys and young men may become the attention

of police or youth offending services as offenders rather than as victims of crime (Pearce et al forthcoming 2009).

As noted above, media representation and resulting public awareness are often 'sold' through combinations of 'sex' and 'slavery'. Provisions and resources in the UK for those who are working in the sex industry are already limited, although there is a history of some service provision including outreach workers, health and social care workers with a few designated services with trained workers specifically targeting women and men working in the sex industry (UKNSWP 2008). These services might identify a case of a woman or young woman who had been trafficked into the country through their outreach and therapeutic resources in local areas. Although some men might be identified through the male sex workers support projects, the gendered expectation that men will be less prone to becoming victims of abuse still dominates and therefore the resources to work with them are more limited (Whowell and Gaffney 2009). A similar pattern emerges within the trafficking discourses, hiding the identification and true numbers of young men who might have been victims of trafficking offences.

Trafficked boys and young men

Harris and Robinson found that the nature of exploitation in 92% of the cases of boys recorded in their data set was unclear. They say that this could be because the boys were smuggled into the UK, rather than trafficked or it could show that the types of exploitation boys are involved in are not as easily identifiable as for girls. For the 11 boys' cases where information regarding the exploitation was given, these included: cannabis cultivation, labour exploitation, begging, and domestic servitude (Harris and Robinson 2007: 6).

In a similar vein, ongoing research identified a young male offender who had been referred to the Youth Offending Team (YOT). The referral to the YOT was made by the police for mobile phone theft. It was not until a relationship was built between the YOT practitioner and the young person involved that the circumstances of the trafficking of the young person became apparent. The case showed that the young person was arrested for stealing mobile phones in one city; they then 'disappeared' to be later rearrested on return after a year away. Following supportive intervention, the young person disclosed a history of having been trafficked into and moved around within the UK. The fact that he had been exploited only emerged following intensive support from the project worker (Pearce et al 2009).

Trafficked girls and young women

Unlike the situation with boys and young men, our knowledge of girls and young women does focus on trafficking for the purpose of sexual exploitation. This means that less is known about other forms of exploitation such as domestic servitude, forced marriage, restaurant work and other forms of labour exploitation. Dowling et al 2007 note that there is a lack of accurate statistics to inform our knowledge of child trafficking into the UK for labour exploitation. They had evidence of trafficking for domestic service, restaurant work and other manual labour, such as work in sweatshops and cannabis factories, credit card and benefit fraud and drug trafficking. The information that is available raises a range of concerns about adequate identification of the problem and appropriate responses to meet the health and social care needs of the women involved.

In the CEOP scoping exercise, of the cases where very high probability of trafficking was involved (level 4 probability), 87% (91) were girls. Of the 91 girls placed in level 4 category of risk:

- Fifty-nine (65%) were trafficked or suspected to have been trafficked for the purpose of sexual exploitation.
- Twenty-one (23%) were trafficked or suspected to have been trafficked for the purpose of domestic servitude.
- The remainder were trafficked or suspected to have been trafficked for purposes of drug trafficking, cannabis cultivation, and other forms of criminal activity, adoption, servile marriages, benefit fraud and other forms of labour exploitation such as working in restaurants (CEOP et al 2007).

Again, similar findings came from a study based in West Sussex, UK, where young women who were identified as victims of commercial sexual exploitation in the UK had been tricked into leaving their county of origin.

> ...we heard that some young women may have been working as prostitutes abroad prior to coming to the UK but are unprepared for the often vicious scenario that awaits them ... the treatment of these women combined with the elements of deception and/or coercion clearly define them as victims of trafficking.
>
> (Harris and Robinson 2007: 83–84)

In summary, these research reports identify the need for the processes of identifying trafficked young people to be better known and understood; for the gendered nature of exploitation to be explored; and for health and social care responses to be improved.

They argue that trafficking cannot be understood as a one-off event but needs to be seen as an ongoing process where a trafficking trajectory is placed in context with previous, current and potential future experiences of violence, poverty and abuse in the country of origin and the country of destination (Pearce et al 2009). A human rights perspective needs to be adopted so that the needs of the individual supersede immigration control. The human right to be listened to and consulted remains as important for interventions with children and young people as it is with adults. This is not only specific for young people trafficked into the country but also for unaccompanied asylum-seeking children (Kohli and Mather 2003, Lane and Tribe 2006).

I want now to explore how both central and local government protocols have been established to try to address some of these issues and suggest ways that work can be developed in the future.

Identification, definition and age dispute

As can be seen from the range of four categories of low to high suspicion of trafficking (CEOP et al 2007), all professional agencies play a role in helping to identify a trafficked young person. As evidenced in other work with very damaged and vulnerable young people, a partnership approach that targets ongoing support during the initial and early stages of engagement is essential to ensure that any protocol can be followed and achieved. The details of the trafficking trajectory will usually only come to light following intensive support and the development of a trusting relationship. This need for a trusting relationship is explored by Hynes (2009) who looks at asylum-seeking individuals' and families' experiences of trust and the impact this has on plans for resettlement. Hynes identifies four forms of trust: social, political, institutional, and restorative trust. She argues that the dispersal system:

> leaves little room for political or institutional trust to be restored and hinders the restoration of social trust
>
> (Hynes 2009: 1)

The trafficking of young people is a substantial, under-reported problem. The methods to identify indicators of trafficking have not yet been incorporated into a range of professional training programmes. As noted, research has been carried out to try to identify the numbers of young people trafficked into the country, including analysis of whether they are trafficked for sexual exploitation or for other forms of exploitation.

A key problem has been on the reliability of data, where figures of trafficked young people are confused with those of separated children (unaccompanied minors or minors with adults who do not have parental responsibility), with smuggled young people or where the signs of trafficking have not been identified by the professional concerned. Indeed, identification may take a long time, evidence suggesting that fear, or language and communication problems, may inhibit a young person from revealing they have been trafficked until years after entry to the country. The pressure to determine the age of the young person at the point of entry to the country can place undue stress at a time when the young person is most in need of reassurance and support.

Using the UN definition of trafficked young people (UN 2003) ECPAT UK with UNICEF produced figures in 2007 predicting that 1.2 million children were suspected victims of trafficking every year. However, it is noted that the recording of information about trafficked young people was poor. The ECPAT report, 'Missing out' noted that:

victim identification was found to be ad hoc, unsystematic and sometimes accidental: information is not always recorded or passed onto relevant agencies; and children might be in the looked after system for some time before they are identified as a victim of trafficking.

(ECPAT 2007: 6)

The scoping exercise carried out by CEOP (2007) also recognised that the identification of trafficked young people was poor, relying much on individual practitioner awareness and expertise. The report noted a gender imbalance where young women were identified, in the main, as having been trafficked for sexual exploitation.

The report noted that identifying cases of trafficking was difficult and that evidence often emerged only years after entry into the country. Different practitioners interpreted 'trafficking' in different ways, and that there were disparate systems with data collection systems which 'lack the capacity to record relevant information about child trafficking' (CEOP et al 2007: 17).

Added to the problem of identification was the problem of young people going missing. Fifty-five per cent of the total 330 suspected cases identified were found to be missing and that if re-found, the young people were reluctant to provide an accurate account of what had happened to them (CEOP et al 2007).

Harris and Robinson (2007) also had problems in confirming the extent and nature of the trafficking of young people in their Pan Sussex study of sexually exploited and trafficked young people. This also identified young people going missing as a serious problem. The report notes that the:

identification of a young person as a victim of trafficking presents very real difficulties at any point in the trafficking process. ... it is rare for the cases to be proven where a young person is intercepted ... there are a number of young people who are identified as being at risk of trafficking who subsequently go missing ... another significant challenge to the identification of trafficking incidents is the young person's lack of awareness of the process they are involved in ...

(Harris and Robinson 2007: 83–84)

Going missing

Research data confirm reports of trafficked young people either going missing shortly after being placed in care or being re-trafficked into the country following deportation (DCSF 2008e: 32). The ECPAT study of 80 cases of suspected trafficked young people showed 60% going missing from local authority care without trace. The CEOP report of 330 cases of suspected trafficked young people noted that 183 (55%) were found to be missing. In a handful of cases, the children were suspected to have been re-trafficked (CEOP et al 2007: 8).

Harris and Robinson found a similar situation in their work in West Sussex (Harris and Robinson 2007). Of the 50 cases of young people who were suspected to have been trafficked, over half went missing within one week of arrival. This reflects concern about the number of unaccompanied minors going missing. Since 2000, 118 UASCs have gone missing from care in West Sussex and over half of these are of suspected trafficking cases.

A further example of six Chinese young women aged 16–17 years highlights similar concerns where trafficking involves the young person 'going missing' within the UK (ECPAT 2007). The young women were stopped at Birmingham Airport on their way to Toronto. Following analysis, it appeared that they had been in the country for up to two years. After being identified at the airport they were placed in different foster care and residential care accommodation. Four of the six then went missing. Another case shows a similar problem where a young woman from Uganda was located by police in 2006, two years after having been brought into the UK for the purpose of commercial sexual exploitation (ECPAT 2007: 20 and 21). As with the Chinese young women, this young woman went missing after being placed in local authority care. Although these cases were identified, it was at too late a stage to protect them from the harm they suffered whilst within the UK. Even after being identified, with details recorded, the young women still then went missing, meaning the disruption of a coherent care plan.

These, and other young people, did not go missing of their own accord. They were abducted, manipulated or coerced by traffickers and traffickers' local networks, showing that trafficking is best understood as a process involving levels of exploitation rather than a one-off event (Pearce et al 2009).

The international traffickers will have contact with 'middle men or women' who will have more detailed knowledge of the country of destination. These 'middle level' operators will have links to the local networks within specific localities where the young people are placed. Like drug markets and other informal global economies, there will be both organised and ad hoc aspects to moving children and young people through international, national and local networks (Ruggiero and Montagna 2008). Research has shown therefore that it is naive to expect the 'rescue' of a child from one stage of the trafficking trajectory to prevent the reoccurrence of further trafficking, even after a period when the child or young person appears to be settled. This means that particularly alert crisis intervention work needs to take place both at the time the young person goes missing and at the time that they return. Police and child protection practitioners need to be able to undertake a rapid assessment of the young person's situation and have resources available to both pursue whatever intelligence is available and offer intensive support to the child.

Delivering this support may not be straightforward as the young person may be unable or unwilling to talk about what has happened to them.

Wall of silence

Another problem in identifying trafficked young people is in how difficult it is to enable them to talk about their experiences. They may be suffering from post-traumatic stress disorder. They may have language and communication difficulties or they may be fearful of talking, being threatened with harm if information about their journey or traffickers is disclosed. The young person might be told by a number of individuals that they are not to talk to anyone. The trafficker may threaten the young person, stopping them from talking to anyone who approached them. A lawyer might advise the young person to remain silent if they are fearful under questioning about their immigration status, and an interpreter might advise them only to talk through certain qualified practitioners. In attempts to build trust with the young person, and in an effort to protect them from further harm, a practitioner may offer advice about who to talk to and when to talk about their circumstances.

This can all create a 'wall of silence' (Pearce et al 2009 forthcoming). The DCSF guidance (2008e) notes a path for practitioners to follow once a suspicion of trafficking has emerged. However, it takes time to enable the young person to feel safe within this process, a feeling of safety being a key component to disclosure.

Child and Adolescent Mental Health Services (CAMHS) have a central role in helping a young person to understand and come to terms with the stress they have experienced. Resources should be available to provide therapeutic and ongoing support to the trafficked young person who may be suffering from a range of mental health problems, including post-traumatic stress disorder. Partnership work between the designated key worker and the CAMHS worker will be essential to support the young person to be able to take advantage of the services available to them. This applies to the provision of other services such as sexual health services and educational services.

Conclusion

The production of the DCSF (2008d) protocol for safeguarding trafficked young people is a step forward in enabling practitioners to identify and work with cases appropriately, but it cannot guarantee that local authorities will be adequately funded to meet the need for interpreters, accommodation support, intelligence gathering and key worker allocation. Research suggests that areas where there are resources specifically targeted towards the needs of vulnerable and socially excluded young people, such as a dedicated projects for sexually exploited children and young people, will be more likely to have a record of identifying trafficked young people. The resource provides a context for workers to share information, and build relevant expertise. Resource, identification and referral then go together, one unlikely to exist without the other.

Despite this comprehensive guidance for Local Safeguarding Children Boards on developing protocols and responding to cases of suspected trafficked young people, there had not been a requirement for data to be collated in a coherent form by the different professional within the local authority that will give evidence of the number of suspected trafficking cases, to record the reason for the trafficking (both the push and the pull reasons), the age of the suspected trafficked child, the country of origin and the nature of their journey into the country. The NRM will, if implemented correctly, begin to address this.

Without a basic recording system that is common to all agencies, we will fail to gain an evidence-based analysis of the scale and nature of the problem. It is clearly not straightforward as, in most cases, the trafficking history only becomes apparent after sustained contact and support work with the young person concerned, and as most traffickers are sophisticated at ensuring that a trafficked young person is hidden from public view. Added to this wall of silence and problem in recording data of cases, there is the fear and reality of the trafficked young people going missing.

In this chapter I have identified some of the problems attached to identifying and defining young people as trafficked. I have noted the need for targeted intervention to prevent the high numbers of young people, both young men and young women, going missing on arrival in the UK. This also identifies the need to address the needs of UK nationals who also go missing and are trafficked internally within the country. However, I have noted caution that different forms of trafficking do not become confused as practitioners' responses will need to vary depending upon the circumstances, knowledge and experience of the young people concerned. In the main I have highlighted that the trafficking of human beings is a process, not a one-off event. As such, it needs to be seen as a part of local, national and international criminal networks, the combating of which rely on good multi-agency work at each level. Finally, I have noted that interventions will need to allow time for a young person to feel confident to talk about their experiences within a trusted and secure relationship. The worry about age disputes needs to be placed in this context, with the welfare, needs and interests of the child taking president.

4 Adolescents in violent partnerships (AVPs): Child abuse and domestic violence?

Introduction

In this chapter I argue that work with sexually exploited young people can learn from some of the policies and practices that have been developed to challenge domestic violence. I propose that the domestic violence experienced by many sexually exploited young people in their interpersonal relationships is not fully appreciated or addressed within many of the child protection interventions that are designed to support them. Indeed, much of the domestic violence experienced by some of the young people in their relationships is understood to be outside the remit of child protection. This chapter reflects on the lessons that have been learnt from work with domestic violence and suggests ways they can inform efforts to safeguard sexually exploited young people.

This is not to attack the work that has developed through safeguarding children boards, or to suggest that child protection should not be the lead initiative in protecting sexually exploited young people. Rather, it is to identify the limitations of child protection policies and procedures that have, in the main, been developed to protect younger children from familial abuse. I refer in this chapter to sexually exploited young people as those who are in their teens, going through puberty and beginning to make the transition from being a child embedded within a family (or care home) to becoming an independent adult functioning autonomously in the public domain. I do not intend to be simplistic here, implying that there can be a chronologic age below or above which a child can cope. Indeed, Chapter 8 refers to the need to look at the young person's developmental, rather than chronological age. What I want to highlight is that traditional approaches within child protection procedures focused on safeguarding from familial abuse might not provide a framework for appropriate responses to meet the needs of many sexually exploited adolescents.

I will develop this argument through four stages.

Firstly, I argue that the resources and expertise available to safeguarding children boards tend to focus on 'child' abuse. This means that there are challenges for safeguarding boards in their aim to protect the older age range of sexually exploited young people.

Secondly, I will look at the way that definitions of domestic violence have focused on interpersonal violence between adults. As such they do not focus on violence experienced by adolescents and young people in their intimate relationships and have therefore, not been referred to in the process of safeguarding young people.

Thirdly, I examine the lessons that we have learnt from work on domestic violence with adults, identifying how they can be applied to safeguarding sexually exploited young people. I refer to some extracts from young people's own dialogue in this section to illustrate the points made.

Finally, I summarise the argument overall, suggesting ways that domestic violence polices and practices can contribute to safeguarding sexually exploited young people.

Child protection and safeguarding sexually exploited young people

Child protection procedures were originally developed to protect children from all forms of abuse. The Children Act 1989 prioritised the welfare of the child as the primary focus for procedures designed to protect children from 'significant harm' (Sections 17 and 20, Children Act 1989). The Children Act of 2004 and the Every Child Matters agenda enforced the importance of good multi-agency work to protect children and support families, aiming for every child and young person to achieve five outcomes, one of which was being safe from harm (DfES 2004a). The safeguarding of sexually exploited children and young people is noted within this outcome, building on the need for all local authorities to follow government supplementary guidance on safeguarding children involved in prostitution (DH 2000).

Despite this broadened agenda, pressure remains on local authority children's services to protect children who are perceived to be the most vulnerable. Coming from a dominant perspective of protecting children within their families, the most vulnerable will invariably be understood as young children experiencing abuse within the home. Enormous developments, prompted by high-profile public enquiries, have taken place to improve the protection of children from familial abuse (Hill 1990). The tragic death of baby P has prompted further enquiries, the outcomes of which are predicted to include an analysis of resource allocation and thresholds for interventions protecting young children from abuse (Community Care 2008, Laming 2009).

The sexual exploitation of young people will, by default, be an additional demand on service delivery. The review of the DH 2000 guidance on safeguarding children involved in prostitution showed 79% of local authorities with protocols for safeguarding sexually exploited children and young people (Swann and Balding 2002). Although the number has increased, and most do now have protocols, we still have some Local Safeguarding Children Boards (LSCBs) without specific subcommittees for safeguarding sexually exploited children and young people.

Research evidence has shown that there are three components to safeguarding sexually exploited children and young people effectively. Areas which do intervene to protect children and young people from sexual exploitation (Lebock and Kink 2006) more successfully tend to have:

- an active protocol;
- a separate active multi-agency subcommittee to safeguard sexually exploited children and young people;
- a dedicated service to follow up the work with the young person concerned (Pearce 2006).

Although there are some local authorities where the three factors co-exist, there is not uniform provision within all local authorities.

As explored in Chapter 2 recent work has produced a sexual exploitation strategy that includes identifying the young people, engaging with them, disrupting and prosecuting the abusers (Jago and Pearce 2008). In authorities where there is not a local pressure group raising the profile of sexual exploitation, where there has not been a high-profile death or murder to prompt the need for dedicated services, where resources are limited and case loads are high, it is not unknown to hear the comment 'we don't have that problem here' (see Chapter 6 for more detail on this).

Although sexual exploitation has become more visible as a social problem, particularly since the concern of abuse via the internet and of the trafficking of young people, services have many other demands, and are therefore extremely stretched. Unless resources are prioritised, it remains peripheral to the safeguarding children board's primary focus on protecting younger children from familial abuse.

Prioritising services and allocating resources are not the only factors at play here. As explored in Part 2, sexually exploited young people can be extremely difficult to identify, to access, engage and maintain contact with. Research and practice in the field has noted that many services for young people are developed and upheld by a few very dedicated and committed practitioners. They persist in developing their services despite funding cuts and despite the 'professional isolation' caused by the continued lack of understanding of the issues they face. However, many other practitioners note that they find work with difficult and demanding adolescents hard to manage (see Chapter 8 for more details).

Unless the practitioner is particularly motivated to work with the young people, they can be quickly discouraged as the young person rejects their support. If the practitioner's case load is already full they may feel it to be legitimate to close the case after a run of missed appointments and rejections. I have referred to this problem in the chapter on therapeutic outreach.

This is particularly apparent if the young person concerned is denying that sexual exploitation is taking place and is asserting their rights to choose how, when and with whom they have a relationship. If the young person is over 16, the age of consent, and is already detached from school and family, the rationale for continuing to keep the case open against other competing demands diminishes.

In work with young people who are sexually exploited through same-sex relationships this is compounded as workers may not feel comfortable with appearing homophobic, being cautious about interfering with the development of a young person's experimentation with gay, lesbian or bisexual orientations. Similarly, a concern with appearing racist may inhibit intervention with young people who are exerting their right to experiment in sexual relationships within the black and minority ethnic (BME) communities (Ward and Patel 2007) (see Chapter 7 for a fuller debate about this). All of these factors can impact on decision-making about case load allocation and case load maintenance.

So, to summarise, while the main drive of the child protection services is directed to protecting children from abuse in the home, and while there is little reward for practitioners to persist in their efforts to engage with sexually exploited young people, services will remain peripheral, marginalised from mainstream delivery.

I turn now to look at how sexually exploited young people have also been 'missed' from the important developments that have taken place within work on domestic violence. I then move to suggesting ways that the lessons we have learnt from work on domestic violence could inform work taking place through safeguarding children boards to protect sexually exploited young people.

Domestic violence

Practice in the field of domestic violence has challenged the physical and emotional abuse of adults in interpersonal relationships. Violence between same-sex couples and violence directed from women to men has been explored, but in the main, the dominant focus has been on interpersonal violence between heterosexual couples, with a male perpetrator and female victim.

The second-wave feminist movement of the 1960s to 1980s made enormous strides in forcing recognition of the prevalence of domestic violence, identifying a split between violence against women in 'female' private places such as the home and violence between men in 'male' public places such as the street, the workplace and pubs and clubs (Stanko 1998).

It was argued that the experiences of women in the home as victims of violence had been overlooked by law enforcement agencies and the impact of violence dramatically under-reported and underplayed. Refuge, the support service established to support victims of violence, opened the first safe house for women and children experiencing domestic violence, in 1971. By 2005 there were over 400 refuges nationally, with 85% of the victims being women (HO 2005). Campaigning and committed work over the last thirty years has raised awareness of these issues, culminating in the need for central government strategies to coordinate efforts against domestic violence.

Recognising the need for a coordinated strategy to tackle domestic violence the government introduced the Domestic Violence, Crime and Victims Act 2004 and the Domestic Violence Action Plan of 2005. Here, domestic violence is described as 'any incident of threatening behaviour, violence or abuse between adults who are or have been in a relationship together, or between family members, regardless of gender or sexuality' (HO 2005: 7). The action plan and other more recent work on domestic violence have acknowledged the importance of a small but important men's movement that is challenging male violence and on developing perpetrator programmes.

Domestic violence between young people

The possibility of domestic violence between children or young people in their girlfriend/boyfriend relationships has not been explored in these debates. Although the 2005 Domestic Violence Action Plan notes that work of the National Society for the Prevention of Cruelty to Children (NSPCC) revealed that too many young people were already subjected to relationship abuse in their teenage years, it does not identify how these young people are to be identified or supported (HO 2005). This is both because young people are, in the main, not expected to be in violent intimate relationships and also because the care and protection of children and young people is expected to be carried out by parents or by substitute care rather than to be the business of adults' domestic violence services.

When children and young people are considered in debates about domestic violence, it is because there is concern about the damage caused to them as witnesses of violence in the home. For example, a survey of Nottingham domestic violence provision showed that at least 750,000 children witness domestic violence every year, and 75% of children on the child protection register have witnessed domestic violence. One-third of the Children's Services caseload at the time involved domestic violence (Nottingham 2005).

However, there is now some emerging recognition that domestic violence does take place between young people in intimate relationships. Research reveals that some young people experienced violence as part of their intimate relationship with their boyfriend or girlfriend, in both same- and opposite-sex relationships. Most of the work on adolescents in violent relationships has been undertaken in the USA. However, more recent work in Scotland and the UK has started to explore what is either called 'adolescent intimate personal violence' (AIPV) or 'teen dating violence'.

The work shows that young people can experience violence within their relationships; that there is a risk of violence in a range of different relationships, including same-sex relationships; and that it can occur within all social strata, not necessarily only within deprived and socially excluded communities. The work from the USA showed that one-quarter of the total 117 young people in same-sex romantic relationships reported partner violence victimisation (Halpern et al 2004) while a study in Scotland reported AIPV from pupils in schools in economically privileged as well as deprived areas (NHS Health Scotland 2005).

Findings from some of these studies have also challenged the clear demarcation between female victim and male perpetrator, suggesting that both young women and young men will expect violence in their intimate relationships and that both are familiar with verbal and physical violence.

For example, the Scottish survey showed that of the students in 10 secondary schools from urban and rural areas who took part in a total of 12 focus groups, between 15% and 20% of both girls and boys reported a range of physical violence. The findings also showed that 2% of girls and 4% of boys reported using violence to try to force a partner to have sex (NHS Health Scotland 2005).

Little is known yet about the extent of AIPV in England. A survey undertaken by the London Borough of Southwark 'Safer Southwark Partnership' showed that 42% of the respondents experienced some form of abusive behaviour from a partner. The survey covered 135 young people from nine different ethnic groups living in 23 different postcode areas. The young people were between the ages of 12 and 24 years, including 74% of respondents aged under 18 years, and 41% of whom were under 16 years old. The study explored the extent of other forms of violence in the lives of those adolescents who are in violent intimate relationships with their partners and friends. It showed that there was a positive correlation between experiencing some form of abusive behaviour and demonstrating behaviour that was abusive (Schutt 2006: 45–46).

The research from the USA has also given us an insight into the impact that the advent of a sexual relationship can have on experiences of violence between teenagers in relationships, suggesting that physical violence is more likely to occur between teenage couples once a sexual relationship has been established. Two surveys showed a correlation between the beginning of sexual activity and the beginning of violence in the relationship. A study of 6548 adolescents aged 12 to 21 years showed that:

> violent victimisation was more likely to occur in romantic relationships that included sexual intercourse, 37% of the respondents reporting sexual relationships experienced at least one form of verbal or physical violence victimisation, compared to 19% of those reporting relationships with no sexual intercourse ... sexual intercourse was significantly more likely to precede violence rather than the reverse
>
> (Kaestle and Halpern 2004: 386)

The second study showed that 78% of adolescents experiencing violence during the 3 months after giving birth had not experienced violence before delivery (Harrikson et al 2002).

These surveys do not imply that sexual activity between young people necessarily results in physical violence, but encourage us to question what happens within interpersonal relationships once a sexual relationship has been established.

These questions must not be looked at uncritically. We need to be mindful of the reasons behind such research, as well as the rigour of the methods used. It could be that liberal and religious beliefs in the USA encourage a focus towards preventing sex between young people, using research findings as a rationale for abstinence. If a baby of a teenage couple is thought to be at risk from its parent's violence, this can be inappropriately used as a rationale for preventing teenagers to become parents by those who are against young people having sexual relationships on moral grounds.

Despite these important questions, the concern raised within research on young people in domestic violent relationships is of how to respond to the young person who is both a partner in a relationship and a child in need of protection. How do we embrace both the adolescent as a potentially responsible partner, or even as a parent, while also recognising the needy child who is being abused within their interpersonal relationships?

A common feature to work with adolescents is in supporting their management of the transition from child to adult. In this process, the young person is negotiating the needs of the child they feel inside them while experimenting in how to become the adult (Coleman and Hendry 1999).

Young people who are in intimate relationships with an abusive partner are facing similar problems that their adult counterpart experiences in a domestic violent relationship. I argue that child protection policies and procedures that are aiming to support adolescents who are in violent relationships can learn from work that has been developed to challenge domestic violence.

I want to continue this now by looking specifically at some lessons from work with domestic violence and explore how they can inform work on safeguarding young people for sexual exploitation. In this next section I will draw on sexually exploited young people's own words to illustrate some of the points I wish to make. Cases referred to are composite, drawing on a range of different case studies, and names are changed to protect confidentiality.

What have we learnt from domestic violence?

Although many lessons have been learnt from work on domestic violence, I identify here four main themes from work with domestic violence that can inform our approach to safeguarding sexually exploited children and young people.

Exploitation is a process, not a one-off event

Research and crime surveys report that domestic violence has long-term negative consequences for those involved. The violence in interpersonal relationships is not a one-off event, but part of an ongoing process within a relationship that may change, go through different stages and structures. If the victim is to leave, it may only be after a long period of time.

The UK British Crime Survey of 2006/07 notes that on average there will have been 35 assaults before the victim calls the police, and an average of two women are murdered every week by a current or former male partner. Research has shown that there are many reasons the violence will not be reported, ranging from social taboo to a lack in confidence in the criminal justice system (Walby and Allen 2004).

Answers to the 'why don't they leave?' question show the complexities of abusive interpersonal relationships, including questions of coercive control, and economic and emotional dependency within the relationship. Rarely, therefore, is the violence, or the leaving home, a one-off event.

Those working with sexually exploited young people have also argued that the exploitation can rarely be understood as a single incident. It is a part of a long, ongoing process where the young person is responding to a number of push and pull factors. As argued in Chapter 5, young people might be pushed into swapping or selling sex because they are wanting to escape poverty, abuse at home or because they feel they have few other alternatives available to support their transition into independent adulthood. Alternatively, or additionally, they might be pulled into swapping or selling sex through coercion by an abusive adult. By encouraging the young person to fall in love with them, the adult uses the young person for financial or other gain.

Rarely is either of these reasons the result of a single incident or event. In the main it is part of a long history of the young person's truancy, running from home, reliance on informal economies, and the related attachments to abusive adults.

I talk more in Chapter 8 about the importance of allowing time with the young person for building a supportive and helpful relationship that will facilitate them in speaking about the problems that they face. Here though, I note that reversing the process of involvement in exploitation can take as long as it has taken for the exploitation of the young person to develop. It might mean reversing the dependency on informal economies for financial survival, which means retraining into education or work. Alternatively, or in addition, it might mean reversing the expectation of abuse within relationships, an expectation resulting from the young person's overriding experience of how relationships work.

For example, when Lorna, aged 17 years, talks of her feelings about her mother who has mental health problems she says:

> Sometimes I wish she was dead. That it is really horrible to wish someone dead but it's how I feel. But she's my Mum. I love her ... It's funny you know that it is really confusing when you really hate somebody and you care for them. That is really bad.

When talking about the relationship that she developed when she was 16 years with a man in his 30s who used her for sex for his friends in return for his drugs she says:

> I know he did all that to me, he was just taking it out on me because I was only 16 and he thought I didn't know lots of things about the world but I did. What he did to me really hurt me, but in a way I don't, but in a way I do forgive him because I love this boy deep down in my heart
>
> (Lorna in Pearce et al 2002)

The man who Lorna was in a relationship with was violent towards her. He repeatedly hit her, abducted her, holding her in his flat for three nights and intimidated her from telling anyone about what was happening.

Not surprisingly, Lorna explains that the mixture she feels between love and hate is 'doing her head in' and that she wanted to remain with her boyfriend, even though she knew he was hurting and exploiting her. She explained that she felt more in control of her situation in her relationship with her boyfriend than she did when at home with her mother.

By the time that Lorna came to the attention of the children's services safeguarding board she was nearly 17 years. She was assessed under Section 17 of the Children Act 1989 that noted her as a child 'in need', but not under Section 20 which would mean that she was to be 'looked after' by the local authority. Discussions took place about what alternative accommodation could be provided to her in light of a shortage of suitable supported housing. This is not uncommon and can often result in young people being placed in bed and breakfast accommodation, despite many of the hotels being located in areas where drug misuse and sex work are evident.

The need for suitable supported accommodation for victims of violence has been fully explored within services for adult victims of domestic violence. Lorna's need for supported accommodation was similar. She received intensive support on a day-to-day level from an allocated worker in the specialist project for sexually exploited children and young people in the borough. This contact was sustained over a two-year period, taking her past her 18th birthday.

Although the project was designed for young people under the age of 18 years, it was recognised that there might be some situations where sustaining contact past the 18th birthday was essential to ensuring longer-term change. This has led a number of projects to consider extending their services to young people beyond the age of 18 years, recognising the time that transition to adulthood can take for some of the young people and the support that they need in accessing and using appropriate services.

During this time Lorna continued to leave and then return to her boyfriend. By the end of the two-year period, a room in supported accommodation had been found and Lorna was beginning to use it, each time staying for longer, building links with housing staff that encouraged her to access a part-time college course. Changes were developing for Lorna over *time*, but it was *time* with a support worker and safe housing that she needed.

Her involvement in sexual exploitation was not a one-off event in her life. It was part of a process that was continued through a supportive and ongoing relationship with a dedicated key worker. The worker herself needed supervision and support to be able to manage Lorna's fluctuating circumstances.

Lorna's situation identifies two points, both already established within discourses of domestic violence. Firstly, leaving a violent partner takes time. It will not happen overnight and will involve repeated episodes of leaving, returning and then leaving again. The victim of the violent relationships needs support throughout each stage of this process. Children's services working with adolescents who are in violent relationships need to be able to tolerate this pattern of behaviour.

Secondly, the process of leaving involves settling into alternative, safe accommodation. While refuges have been developed to meet the needs of adult victims of domestic violence, we have little supported housing that is fully equipped to manage fluctuating behaviour of the victim and the associated violence they experience. Children's services need support in considering how this service can be developed in the future.

Relationship-based interventions: The independent specialist advisor

Building from this, we can see the significance that a positive relationship with a professional can have for a sexually exploited young person. One of the key developments in work with domestic violence is the creation of independent domestic violence advisor (IDVA) posts. These appointments provide 'dedicated advice and assistance from an independent source, available to those inside and outside the criminal justice system' (HO 2005: 9). The evidence for the need for these posts came from a systematic evaluation of 27 domestic violence projects (HO 2005), and from work focused on evaluating support to victims of violence (Hester and Westmarland 2005). Evidence showed that a relationship with a dedicated worker helped those in violent relationships to address their situation over time. The dedicated worker would continue support even if the violent relationship continued, would accompany the victim through all police investigations and at court procedures if the case was taken forward. Seven key factors that needed to be addressed in the appointment of the IDVA were identified. The post holder needs to be:

- Independent from police services.
- Professional, not allowing an untrained volunteer to hold responsibility for complex cases.
- Fully aware of safety issues facing those working with or experiencing domestic violence, including the need for safe accommodation and safe relationships.
- Trained in crisis intervention.
- Able to undertake risk assessments that evaluate risks:
  - of potential harm to themselves in their work;
  - of harm to the victim of violence – both in terms of the risks faced by staying within the violent relationship and in leaving.
- Aware of and able to manage partnership work taking place within multi-agency interventions.
- Able to identify clear aims and outcomes in their work (HO 2005: 10).

Before exploring how the IDVA initiative is applicable to supporting sexually exploited young people, I will use work with Nina to illustrate some of the points I am making here.

Contact between Nina and the dedicated sexual exploitation project in the local area had lasted while Nina was aged between 15 and 18 years. During this time she repeatedly left and returned to her violent partner. Faced with the frustration that there is no one rescue operation that would prevent Nina from continuing her relationship with her boyfriend, the sexual exploitation project workers' main focus was on supporting her to keep returning to the project. It was to engage her in activities that would help build self-esteem in the times that they saw her, and on helping her to express her feelings about her boyfriend.

Project workers were concerned that as well as being violent, Nina's boyfriend had persuaded her to have sexual relationships with his friends. He was a heroin user and was known locally to work as a pimp. Over the three-year period Nina managed to sustain some attendance at school. She fluctuated between living at home and staying with her boyfriend and, most importantly, continued to attend drop-in sessions and one-to-one meetings with the local sexual exploitation project staff.

On one occasion when Nina had been badly attacked by her boyfriend she attended the project and wrote down the reasons that she was going to return to his flat. She was returning because:

- She has had a miscarriage with his baby and she wants to tell him so he knows how much she has suffered.
- She thinks that if she stays with him for long enough she can change him – make him treat her differently.
- If she leaves him before the police can do anything her family may suffer.
- He is dependant upon her, needing her for money for his drugs.

(Pearce et al 2009)

Much of this language is common to domestic violence cases. Nina wanted her boyfriend to realise how he had hurt her; she was aware that he was threatening her family as well as herself but most importantly, she felt that if she managed to stay with him, he would, over time, treat her better. This sense of waiting for things to improve is not uncommon. What is more unusual is that these feelings were those of a 16 year old, rather than of an adult in a violent relationship. Nina needed support to see that other more positive and caring relationships were possible, and that she had the potential to engage in different activities outside of her relationship. This took time. Eventually Nina accepted appropriate independent accommodation, took a part-time job while returning to study and worked with project staff to successfully take a case out against her former boyfriend for abduction.

One of the successes of the work with Nina was her continued contact with the project staff who understood sexual exploitation, and were able to advocate for Nina in her contact with her family and with other professionals such as police, social workers and education staff. Referring back now to the list of requirements for the IDVAs, we see similar requirements. The project worker was independent, based in a local project with links to, but functioning separately from, police or social services. They were professionally trained, with a thorough knowledge of youth work, child protection, sexual and mental healthcare and of the role of the police and legal system.

As with IDVAs, undertaking risks assessments is central to the work, particularly when needing to explain boundaries on confidentiality to the young person so that a risk of 'significant harm' results in their situation being reported to the safeguarding board.

Similarly, crisis intervention is an often overlooked but essential part to work with sexually exploited children and young people. As Howe (1998) has argued, young people can create chaos and crisis around themselves as a means of avoiding contact with a worker who might be asking them to address their difficult situation. Many sexually exploited young people will be responding to crisis in their lives and also creating (albeit unconsciously) crisis as a means of avoiding unbearable circumstances. Howe goes on to argue that it is an ongoing relationship with a trained and reliable adult that can begin to address such chaos, a relationship that domestic violence practice has endorsed as important within the IDVA initiative.

The IDVA initiative also means that the post holder is available to give advice and support to other professionals about domestic violence. As noted above, children's services, child protection workers and police may not have the time or the resources to reach out to and protect sexually exploited children and young people who may remain 'invisible' to mainstream service providers. Work from a number of specialist sexual exploitation projects across the country shows that in addition to acting as advocates for individual young people, they play an important role in training local health, education and social work staff about sexual exploitation.

As seen in Chapter 3, this is even more apparent in work with young people who have been trafficked for the purpose of sexual exploitation. Dedicated and trained posts for supporting sexually exploited young people over time, supporting them through court if appropriate and raising awareness about the nature of sexual exploitation within the area is essential for the aims of Every Child Matters 2004 to be achieved.

Specialist courts: A comprehensive, inclusive provision

The centrepiece of the National Domestic Violence Delivery Plan (HO 2005) has been the continued expansion of the Specialist Domestic Violence Court (SDVC) programme. The SDVC is not a building or physical representation of a court but is a concept; one that puts a multi-agency approach at the centre of improving criminal justice outcomes in domestic violence cases and that provides scope to 'cluster' cases together and 'fast track' them through the court process. The specialist court programme is a coordinated community response to domestic violence that combines both criminal justice interventions (e.g. dedicated domestic violence prosecutors) and non-criminal justice interventions (e.g. the IDVA posts). The specialist domestic violence courts recognise the significance of the urgency to progress a case when a victim is ready to prosecute, to provide a dedicated support (IDVA as above) and to educate those in the legal system about the nature and extent of violence. This is to ensure that the court process supports the victim and the sentencing patterns reflect the seriousness of the crime. The specialist domestic violence courts aim to create close coordination between different professionals, with key individuals identified and held to account for the delivery of their section of the service system.

Evaluation of their effectiveness noted three key positive benefits of SDVCs and Fast Track Systems (FTSs) showed that:

- Both 'clustering' and 'fast-tracking' domestic violence cases enhances the effectiveness of court and support services for victims.
- Both SDVC and FTS arrangements make advocacy and information sharing easier to accomplish.
- Victim participation and satisfaction is improved and thus public confidence in the criminal justice system is increased.(Cook et al 2004: 4)

The evaluation of 216 cases involving domestic violence at the early stages in the magistrate's court found that all courts showed value for money. Significant financial savings were noted if domestic violence is tackled early, such as reduced retractions, healthcare savings and complementing social service monitoring of children (HO 2006c: 12).

There was also some evidence of increased guilty pleas from perpetrators when victims were supported and, in some courts, an increase in late guilty pleas. While early pleas are always preferable, late guilty pleas can also be seen as a successful outcome as defendants often try to 'string out' the court process expecting the victim to withdraw (www.crimereduction.homeoffice.gov.uk/domesticviolence/domesticviolence59.htm).

The DH 2000 guidance for safeguarding children involved in prostitution noted dual aims. One was to protect young people and the other was to prosecute abusers. While there have been developments to meet the former aim, we are lagging behind in knowing how to gather credible evidence, support victims through the court process and increase conviction rates (Jago and Pearce 2008). There has been very little use of the legislation available in the Sexual Offences Act 2003. Although alternative legislation such as the Abduction Act 1984 has occasionally been used, there is shamefully little happening to ensure that those who sexually exploit children and young people are disrupted, challenged and prosecuted.

The SDVC is an example of how this could be done. It could inform the attempt to challenge the sexual exploitation of young people. The SDVC has 11 core components. Components 1 to 3 already exist in the guidelines for safeguarding children involved in prostitution (DH 2000). These are that each local authority should have: (1) multi-agency partnerships with protocols; (2) multi-agency risk assessment conferences; and (3) multi-agency public protection arrangements. Indeed, Jago and Pearce's (2008) work supported the suggestion that police sexual exploitation services could helpfully be placed in public protection units.

However, components (4) specialist support services; (5) trained and dedicated criminal justice staff; (6) court listing considerations; (8) data collection and monitoring; and (9) court facilities, are not specific requirements for subcommittees of safeguarding children boards.

We know that in local authorities where specialist projects do exist and where data on sexually exploited children and young people are collected and recorded in annual reports (see Sheffield 2007 and Awaken Project 2007a for examples) it is possible to gain an overview of the scale of the problem, the amount of cases that have been taken to court and the outcomes of convictions. However, this data collection is the exception rather than the rule. As explored in Chapters 1 and 2 much more has to be done to collate evidence of, and data about, sexual exploitation. Drawing on two of the remaining components to the SDVCs, I look now at where innovative developments could take place to improve services for sexually exploited young people.

Equality and diversity

The seventh component to the SDVC is to address equality and diversity. This notes findings from the evaluation that:

> There is a paucity of data in relation to ethnicity and disability, which are poorly recorded by most CJS agencies working with the courts evaluated here and noted in research elsewhere. Also noted was a lack of awareness of issues around same sex relationships both in relation to the processing of domestic violence cases and in terms of domestic violence support (which is geared primarily to male on female abuse). There are significant problems around access to translation and interpreting services – for the police, the courts and in the wider support community.
>
> (HO 2006c: 12)

The SDVC manual includes information on the role of agencies in overcoming barriers for BME victims. It provides information on BME-related advice services and on services for male victims of domestic violence (HO 2006c: annex 3 to 10).

The issue of extending services to BME communities has been noted in many evaluations of domestic violence services, both in the UK and the USA (Riger et al 2002).

The same has been argued for work with sexually exploited children and young people. The overriding assumption, reflecting theories of gendered power relations, is that the victim of exploitation will be female and the perpetrator male (Palmer 2001, Lillywhite and Skidmore 2007). Also, although some members of BME communities are sexually exploited, it has been argued that they have poor access to support projects.

There has been concern about identifying one particular culture as either vulnerable to exploitation or likely to exploit children and young people. For these reasons, the engagement with the BME communities on issues of sexual exploitation has been poor and many exploited young people are unsupported in their efforts to challenge the abuse (Ward and Patel 2007). I want now to refer to a case that explores these issues in more detail (see Pearce et al 2009 forthcoming).

Tom is of African Caribbean origin, living with his mother who is separated from Tom's father and in a current relationship with a violent partner. Tom was aged 15 years when he was referred to the Youth Offending Team (YOT) after police were called to an incident where Tom had attacked his mother's boyfriend in self-defense. Tom is gay and his partner, Mike, aged 36 years, 'keeps an eye' on Tom.

Mike, a white British man, is very controlling and there was concern that Mike encouraged Tom to have sexual relationships with other older men. Mike is overprotective, keeping Tom in his sight as much as possible. Tom understands Mike to be looking after him, distracting him from any further offending behaviour, bringing him to appointments with the YOT.

Mike is saying that once Tom has his 16th birthday, he will take him abroad and help him start a new life, away from the court and away from his family.

It is not uncommon for YOTs to receive referrals of black young men to their case load. Indeed, research evidence shows that black young people are over-represented in the criminal justice system (Coleman and Brooks 2009).

What is unusual, is for the sexual relationship between Mike and Tom to be identified and referred to a specialist sexual exploitation project in the area. It happened in this case because the specialist project had run training with the YOT to identify 'early warning signs' of sexual exploitation, and because there was good multi-agency work taking place on the LSCB subcommittee for sexually exploited young people.

Mike's controlling and violent behaviour made it very difficult for the sexual exploitation project to meet with Tom, and joint work between them and the YOT was necessary to secure a time and place to meet. However, over time Tom was introduced to a male sexual health worker and was put in touch with a support service for black gay young men. He began to confront his acceptance of violence and to challenge some of Mike's restricting and controlling behaviour. Without such multi-agency work, Tom's needs might not have been met and he might have continued to offend.

Such cases encourage us to challenge the dominant assumptions that sexual exploitation takes place within heterosexual relationships. They also ask us to consider the impact of race and racism on our service delivery. The LSCB subcommittees for sexually exploited children and young people are not required to report on how many cases are taken to court, or on how actions of the perpetrators have been disrupted and challenged. Neither do they have to report on how they are reaching out to sexually exploited young men and young people from the BME communities. The 11 components of the SDVCs do require actions on these points. This could be used as a strong example of how services for sexually exploited young people could be improved.

Perpetrator programmes

Component (11) of the SDVCs notes the need for community-based perpetrator programmes to be developed. It asks for information to be widely available on perpetrator programme publications and resources; on key standards for perpetrator programmes outside of the criminal justice system and on the potential risks of running perpetrator programmes.

Practice suggests that the young people and those who sexually exploit them often know one another through local networks.

For example, it is not uncommon for young people to bring other young people into exploitative situations. Helen, a 15-year-old young woman attacked her girlfriend 'Sue' because Sue was starting to have a relationship with Helen's ex-boyfriend. All three were living on an inner city housing estate where low-level drug crime was prevalent. Steve lived in a flat which was a meeting place for young people truanting from school. Local concern was that young people were exchanging sex in the flat for drugs and alcohol.

Helen had considered Steve to be her boyfriend but left the relationship after Steve attacked her whilst holding her in his flat for three days and nights. Helen had introduced Sue, a friend from school, to Steve who then became Sue's boyfriend. Helen could see Sue, her friend, starting a relationship with Steve and could not persuade her to stop seeing him so took her anger and fear out on Sue directly, beating her up.

Not only do the young people on the estate know of the flats and other locations where informal economies exist, but so do the adults who engage with the young people. These 'closed networks' serve as endorsement of the activities taking place, giving their own rationales and explanations for what is happening, which make them feel and appear acceptable. In these networks young women may become aware that they can exchange sex for drugs, accommodation or money. Young people will become aware that they can exploit others for their own gains. Apart from some work led by Barnardos and some relationship and sex education in Personal, Social, Health and Economic Education initiatives in schools (ww.barnardos.co.uk – school pack) little if any work has taken place in challenging boys' and young men's assumptions of and involvement with sexual exploitation. Similarly, while sex offender programmes with adult men have developed, there is still much development to be done to challenge dominant attitudes of men who sexually exploit young people.

The point here is twofold.

Firstly, it endorses the need for local support work on estates and in specific localities to enable young people to talk about their knowledge of who the perpetrators are, where they live, who they associate with and how they access and use young people.

Secondly, it endorses work on domestic violence that has shown that many perpetrators of the violence can want to challenge their behaviour. Men's groups and other specialist agencies have developed ways of supporting perpetrators to try to change their behaviour and break the pattern of violence. This approach could be considered in work with sexually exploited young people, trying to engage local perpetrators known to the young people to address their behaviour. This does not mean condoning exploitation and abuse. It means drawing on how police and perpetrator programmes have worked together and using this knowledge in attempts to disrupt and prosecute abusers (see www.respect.co.uk for further details).

Some important work has been carried out to evaluate perpetrator programmes, arguing for their continuation and development as an essential part of any strategy designed to improve safety within interpersonal relationships (Dobash and Dobash 2000, 2005). In her evaluation of service provision for perpetrators of violence in one local authority, Hester (2006: 3) notes that:

> some perpetrators had not tried to find help to stop being violent because they did not accept that their behaviour was a problem. ... Others only began to accept that their behaviour was a problem once they had been convicted and sent on a probation-led programme ...

But that:

> ... for some men, domestic violence perpetrator programmes had clearly had a major impact on the way they managed all inter-personal relationships, not only those with their partners
>
> (page 4)

She concludes, noting that:

> Specialist services are needed for some groups, such as young men ...
>
> (page 4)

Some work has been carried out in the USA exploring the profile of the adolescent male perpetrator of dating violence, concluding that there are similarities with young men who commit other offences. The work suggests that teen boys who abuse their dating partners are more likely to have experienced child abuse or neglect, witnessed domestic violence and to use alcohol or drugs than their non-abusive counterparts. The work also notes that young men who abuse their dating partners are more likely to have sexist attitudes supporting male domination over females and are more likely to associate with peers that support these attitudes (Peacock and Rothman 2001).

Conclusion

This chapter argues that work with sexually exploited children and young people must remain within the child protection/safeguarding agenda, but that it can learn from strategies developed to understand and support adults who are experiencing domestic violence. This means safeguarding boards being open about their limitations to protect older teenagers who are in domestic violent situations. In particular it means recognising that, as with domestic violence, sexual exploitation is not a one-off event that young people can be 'rescued' from, but behaviours that need long-term interventions to identify and engage with. Change can and does happen, but not over night and not without long-term support.

There is a need for dedicated specialist and trained staff to work with the young people concerned, following the model as developed for IDVAs. Also, we need better means of gathering evidence that can be used to take a case against an abuser and more sophisticated and supportive court environments. The SDVC provides a model of how this could be achieved in processing cases against abusers.

Finally, we need to develop a greater awareness of the need to support young people who might themselves go on to sexually exploit others, raising the profile of these issues in preventative work in schools and on active perpetrator programmes for those convicted. This way we will be able to begin to respond to the complex and ongoing needs of young people who fall outside the traditional approaches developed with children's services for protecting younger children from familial abuse.

Part 2

5 Risk and resilience

I'm on a health and beauty course at college now. I didn't see myself as vulnerable to being used sexually but to drug use, because of the area where I live, loads of kids use smack. ... I went out with Jim to get at this girl that I didn't like. I knew what I was doing, but now I feel used by him ... You should talk to Kath. She's vulnerable, very. She's stupid, she sleeps with the lads for fags and drink, you know. That's why I lost it with her the other night and now I'm being done for GBH.

(Helen, aged 15, in Pearce et al 2002: 47)

It's when you don't know your choices that other people have all the power

(Nicola, aged 17, NSPCC 2004, service user)

Introduction

There are a number of things evident within both of these quotes above. Helen is not presenting as a vulnerable victim groomed into abuse. Indeed, she felt that she was more vulnerable to problem drug use than to sexual exploitation. This does not deny that grooming is not a risk, but presents a different account of vulnerability in this particular situation. Each and every person understands and defines their own vulnerabilities in different ways depending upon a range of issues including their self-awareness, their previous experiences of abuse and their current attachments, strengths and confidences. That is, individual risks and resiliencies cannot be generalised. Helen also recognises the shift from the time when she wanted a relationship with Jim, an older man on her estate who encouraged girls to sleep with his friends, to a later time where she feels used by him. She knows her estate and friends well. She is aware that Kath is vulnerable to exploitation and wants to do something about this. The only way that she felt able to stop Kath from becoming further exploited was to challenge her outright, a challenge that resulted in a fight which got out of hand.

Helen's words illustrate an awareness of different people's individual risk factors (*she's vulnerable, very*), of environmental risk factors (*because of the area where I live, loads of kids use smack*), of an understanding of abuse (*I feel used by him now*), and an attempt to be resilient against adversity (*I'm on a health and beauty course now*).

Nicola is demonstrating a clear understanding of the relationship between vulnerability, knowledge, choice and power. Without knowledge of your choices, you cannot act and therefore you are vulnerable to those who have the power. In her eyes, knowledge of choice brings power. She later went on to explain that it was through involvement with the dedicated project for sexually exploited young people that she began to learn about other choices available to her and, therefore, began to feel more powerful, less vulnerable and less at risk.

In this chapter I draw on young people's experiences to identify some of the risks that can be faced by sexually exploited children and young people. I also look at some of the resilience factors that can equip them to avoid, withstand or minimise the impact of the harm. In so doing, I consider whether risk assessment models can help us to identify how to protect and support young people in their transition towards adulthood. I do this by questioning the motivation to protect young people: is it driven by a desire to divert them from harm or from behaviour that offends moral sensitivities? With this question in mind, I explain the definition of sexual exploitation that has been developed to encompass the full range of risks that young people might face and refer to a model risk assessment framework for protecting the young people concerned.

Risk aware or risk adverse

Before I move to look at the issues raised above, I want to add a word of caution. Gill (2007) argues that we are running the risk of becoming so 'risk averse' that we aim to protect all young people from all harm, dramatically reducing their capacity to build resilience and to learn to cope with the inevitable pains of tragedies that do befall all of us at some point in childhood, adolescence and adult life. Cooper and Lousada (2005) argue that the recent focus on monitoring, assessing and accounting for risk is in itself a defense, an attempt to protect ourselves from the inevitable emotional pains that life throws our way.

Are we increasingly becoming a society that is unduly focused on developing strict and rigid structures for 'risk management', in some cases with an ultimate (and yet impossible) aim of eradicating all risk (Beck 1992, Adam et al 2000)? Also, while we focus on the damages that can be done to young people, are we denying them the opportunity to celebrate their achievements?

While adolescence is associated with risks such as teen smoking, high suicide rates, binge drinking, and high teenage conception rates, there is an alternative story that focuses on how such problems can mask a more positive picture of resilient youth (Sharland 2005). Less advertised data show alternative stories of declining conception rates, albeit they are still the highest in Europe, increasing numbers of young people in education and employment (Coleman and Scofield 2007) and of young people more likely to be victims, rather than perpetrators, of crime (Goldson et al 2002). Indeed, Rutherford (1986) shows us that risk taking is part and parcel of the dynamic of growing up, and that media and political responses might over-sensationalise risk-taking behaviour, begging the question why young people are, and have been, through generations, so demonised as 'risky' (Pearson 1983).

It is important to bear these points in mind as we move to look at the questions of risk and resilience amongst sexually exploited children and young people.

Identifying the risk of sexual exploitation

One concern expressed by practitioners and young people themselves is that a focus on the risk of them becoming sexually exploited is a confused response to fears that young people may be sexually active.

It is not sexual activity per se that I am arguing we need to protect young people from; but rather the risks that are associated with relationships with abusive adults who do not have the young person's welfare at heart. This means that we need to become better equipped at helping the young person to be aware of the dangers they can face in relationships and improve ways of disrupting and prosecuting those who do abuse the young people.

Many young people have happy and healthy sexual relationships in an age-appropriate manner (Moore and Rosenthal 2006). As I note in a previous work (Pearce 2007a, 2007b) this is not to say that there are no risks for sexually active young people, particularly younger adolescents. Longitudinal studies have noted a positive association between problem drinking, marijuana use and delinquent behaviour (school truancy, antisocial behaviour and offending behaviour) and early sexual intercourse (Jessor et al 2003). The National Survey of Sexual Attitudes and Lifestyle (NATSAL) found that up to 50% of sexually active young people under the age of 16 years used no contraception and regretted that it happened so early in their life (Wellings 2001). From a questionnaire survey of 7395 13- and 14-year-old school pupils, Wight et al (2000) found that 18% of boys and 15.4% of girls had experienced sexual intercourse and felt regretful that it had happened.

In both studies, the regret was related to feelings of control within their sexual relationship; the young men saying that they lacked control within their peer groups as they had responded to peer pressure to have sex and to exert control over the young women, pressurising them into sexual intercourse. The young women felt that they lacked control: saying that they found it hard to say no and worried that they would loose the boyfriend if they did not have sex.

The lack of perceived control has been shown to be an indicator of low self-esteem and low self-worth, both of which can undermine a young person's healthy sexual development (Aggleston et al 2000). Irrespective of the age of the young person, a number of studies have shown teenagers first become sexually active when under the influence of alcohol or drugs.

Wight et al (2000) found from their study of teenagers, that 39% of young women and 40% of young men said that they were 'drunk or stoned' the first time that they had sexual intercourse. The sexual activity was not always desired. Coleman and Cater (2005) found that from a sample of 39 interviewees aged 14 to 17 years who had sexual experiences while drunk, 32 regretted the activity. Also, the work showed that drunkenness could result in an inability to control or recognise a potentially risky situation.

Similarly, few young people had contact with the sexual health services that they needed. Coleman and Scofield (2005: 69) reported that many young people do not know of sexual health services in their area where they can access support.

While these generic risks are associated with unwanted sexual activity amongst young people, it is the dangers presented by abusive relationships that need specific attention. While this distinction is usually maintained, some discourses can slip into generalised assumptions that it is sexual activity, rather than abusive relationships, that is the key focus. It is important that caution is applied to prevent this from happening as sex, rather than the nature of an abusive relationship can become the focal point for concern, raising anxiety about sexual activity rather than about the emotional and psychological welfare of the young person concerned.

An example illustrates this point. A 14-year-old young woman, Jo, had been held in police protection late one evening. She needed this protection as she had been picked up from the street by police after having been reported missing by her care home. She was on her own in central London, drunk and lost.

She spoke to the researcher she met after this incident about how she used risky sexualised behaviour as a way of attracting attention to herself. She felt that her own needs, and the loss that she felt having been removed from her family home after she disclosed sexual abuse from her father, had not been recognised or worked with. She said that she 'shagged 26 blokes in seven months', that she 'wasn't worried about AIDS' and that she will 'return to this if I am not allowed to go home to live with my mum'.

It was evident that there were genuine problems experienced by her mother in being able to care appropriately for Jo. Her home environment presented dangers that meant it was not safe for her to return. However, she felt that this had not been fully explained and she still felt confused about why she was separated from her mother. She was returned to her residential care home where she had not yet been allocated a key worker. Her relationship with children's services was not strong as she had experienced two changes of social workers in the previous year, and, because she felt let down by staff who had left before, she was slow to engage with her new worker.

Jo was referred to a sexual health clinic which had resources to address her sexual health needs but not her emotional and relationship based needs. Her feelings of loss, abandonment and fear of her future were, she felt, not being addressed and she continued to use sex as a way of drawing attention to her circumstances. In this instance, although her sexualised behaviour was creating health risks, it was the sexual health and physical health needs that were being responded to rather than her concerns about her emotional wellbeing. The point here is that sex, and the anxiety it can create, can unduly become the focus of a risk assessment, leaving the emotional and mental health risks facing the young person unnoticed.

I want to take this relationship between risk, resilience and sexual exploitation a little further in this chapter as while there are some risks associated with sexual activity, it is the context within which the sexual activity occurs that needs assessing and responding to. I argue that while it is helpful to be clear about the risks that face young people concerned, we should not focus on 'risk' at the cost of excluding 'resilience'. As it is important to be able to protect young people from undue risk, it is also important to help them to build their resiliencies to danger and to support them in developing their own protective factors for longer-term self-help, agency and self-determination.

Firstly, it is helpful to be clear about what is meant by risk and then to explore some of the key components to those risks faced by sexually exploited children and young people. Next, I will look at the relationship between risk and resilience before moving to explore how risk assessments can support young people to build protective factors so that they can play a key role in their own movement away from further harm or abuse.

To explore this further I look at how 'risk' itself has been defined and understood and then look at its relationship with resilience in more detail, focusing on the meaning this can have to our work with sexually exploited children and young people.

Applying the concept of risk to sexual exploitation

Coleman and Hagel (2007: 2) provide a helpful breakdown of four ways that the concept of risk can be applied to young people.

- Risk factors: the term that usually refers to the factors that might contribute to poor outcomes for young people, such as poverty, deprivation, illness or dysfunctional family background.
- Young people at risk: this term is used to refer to those who are potentially vulnerable, such as those who are socially excluded, those who are subject to abuse or neglect, and those who are in custody or in care.
- Risk behaviour, or risky behaviour: this term applies to potentially harmful behaviour that young people might engage in, such as having unsafe sex, abusing substances such as illegal alcohol or illegal drugs, or taking part in antisocial activities.
- Young people who pose a risk to society: this concept is used to apply to those who engage in antisocial behaviour or who in other ways pose a threat to their communities.

Sexually exploited children and young people have been a focus within each of these four categories of risk. Research and practice have highlighted a number of 'risk factors' that are seen to place young people at risk of sexual exploitation, and certain young people have been seen to be particularly 'at risk' of exploitation (Harper and Scott 2005). Young people's sexualised *risky beha-viours* have been of concern to practitioners working on sexual exploitation (Scott and Skidmore 2006). The use of antisocial behaviour orders and the provision of the final 'opt-out' clause in the government guidance (DH 2000) allowing prosecution for offences relating to prostitution identify the punitive policy framework that can be used when sexually exploited young people are seen to be posing *a risk to society*. Indeed, the report from the London Assembly's Safer London Committee on 'Street prostitution in London' recommended a review of the use of antisocial behaviour orders for those selling sex (London Assembly 2005). As said above, these different forms of risk cannot be seen in isolation from resilience. I give a brief overview of some of the ways that risk and resilience have been understood before moving on to look at specific impact of risk and resilience on the assessment of sexually exploited children and young people's needs.

Applying the concept of resilience to sexually exploited young people

Resilience has been defined as the capacity to transcend adversity (Rutter 1985). The more resilient the young person, the more they are able to draw on their own resources to overcome difficult conditions (Gilligan 1999).

> Resilient children are better equipped to resist stress and adversity, cope with change and uncertainty, and to recover faster and more completely from traumatic events or episodes
>
> (Newman 2002: 2)

Newman goes on to argue that while exposure to certain risk factors might increase the probability that children will experience poor outcomes, resilient factors will conversely increase the likelihood that children will be able to 'resist or recover from the exposure to adversity' and the 'successful management of risk is a powerful resilience – promoting factor in itself' (Newman 2002: 3).

It is possible to help young people to develop their resilience, not specifically by protecting them from all risks or adversities, but by helping them to learn to judge what is possible for them to manage. This means being able to create a situation where the young person can be encouraged to understand the risks that they face and consider how much they themselves can cope with.

There are, as Rutter (1985) explains, delicate balancing acts to be performed when helping young people to develop resilience to adversity. This involves helping them to change their exposure to risk, to interrupt a chain reaction of negative events (one bad thing leading to another), to establish and maintain self-efficacy and self-esteem and to create opportunities for change (Rutter 1985). Newman develops this further by arguing that interventions with young people need to be focused on how to support young people to build their resi-liencies. The more resilient the young person, the more they can access their own protective factors to help them to overcome adversity.

The successful management of risk is a powerful resilience – promoting factor in itself

(Newman 2002: 3)

Risk and resilience: A partnership

It is argued that risk and resilience are best understood as working in partnership. As noted by Newman and Blackburn (2002: 3):

> risk factors heighten the probability that children will experience poor outcomes. Resilience factors increase the likelihood that children will resist or recover from exposure to adversity. Positive child development is not simply a matter of reducing or eliminating risk factors and promoting resilience. The successful management of risk is a powerful resilience-promoting factor in itself

Coleman and Hagel (2007) continue this train of thought, noting four main points from a review of literature about the relationship between risk, resilience and adolescence.

- Firstly, they note that there is strong evidence from longitudinal studies that where there are protective factors available, children and young people do recover from short-term adversity – enabling the majority of children and young people to have the capacity for being resilient to some adversity when the risk factors are limited.
- Secondly, that where risk factors are continuous and severe, only a minority can cope as the more serious the adversity, the stronger the protective factors need to be.
- Thirdly, resilience can only develop through exposure to risk, through contact with what Rutter (1985) calls 'steeling experiences'.
- Finally, and most importantly, for work with sexually exploited children and young people:

> the major risk factors for children tend to lie within chronic and transitional events, rather than in the acute risks. Thus children show greater resilience when faced with acute adversity such as bereavement, or short-term illness, and less resilience when exposed to chronic risks such as continuing family conflict, long-term poverty and multiple changes of home and school

(Coleman and Hagel 2007: 14)

It is not the one-off incident that might damage the young person's longer-term ability to cope; it is the ongoing, somewhat relentless experience of abuse, rejection, change and instability that impacts negatively on the young person's capacity to manage, to be resilient. However, as will be argued below, one of the lessons from research is that it is never too late. The fact that the young person might have experienced a history of abuse and is continuing to place themselves in risky and dangerous relationships need not be a reason for failing to intervene. Protective factors can be developed, albeit with the need for longer-term, supported intervention addressing both individual, familial and environmental factors.

It is argued that a method of enabling this is through giving the young person some control in dealing with their problems. Protective factors are enhanced by:

> the promotion of self efficacy and self esteem through enabling children to exert agency over their environment
>
> (Newman 2002: 5)

Young people need to be encouraged to identify and draw on some of the benefits of their actions and to take control over their environment themselves:

> *a key protective factor for children who have experienced severe adversities is the capacity to recognise any **benefits** that may have accrued, rather than focusing solely on negative effects, and using these insights as a platform for affirmation and growth.*
>
> (Newman 2002: 5, italics in text)

Risk, resilience and relationship-based thinking

Newman (2002, 2004) has shown that where adversities are continuous and severe and where protective factors are absent, young people are less resilient and less able to recover from trauma or distress. However, even in these circumstances, there are still opportunities to build a young person's resilience. Resilience is dynamic, having the capacity to emerge later in life after earlier periods of coping problems. Research from the US and UK show that if the individual young person can be encouraged to be active and independent, and can be supported by a caring adult, resilience can be enhanced. In other words, it is not too late to provide protective factors for adolescents whose earlier childhoods might have been disrupted.

To put this into effect means allocating resources towards helping the young person concerned to build constructive relationships. This relationship-based thinking approach to the work builds on the idea that, even if poor attachments have been experienced at an earlier stage in the young person's life resulting in them having a vulnerable and insecure sense of self, it is still possible for the young person to be helped to form other 'good' attachments and to begin to develop a stronger, more secure 'inner world' (Howe 2005).

For the young person to have access to a reliable adult who can hear their needs and continue to 'be there' and 'hold them in mind' will give them confidence to:

- Believe that it is possible for someone to value them, to see them worthy of time and effort.
- Experience a model of a non-abusive, good relationship that can be copied and reproduced in interactions with others.

'Being there' for the young person reassures them that a relationship can be strong enough to withstand the pain and trauma that they might have experienced. It means providing a non-judgemental framework from which they can start to reflect on some of their behaviours. This does not mean providing a relationship without boundaries, tolerating unacceptable behaviour from the young person without critique. It means clarifying what constitutes a caring relationship, asking for recognition of this and continuing to work at establishing it, even if there are gaps where the young person goes missing, runs away from it, is difficult and abusive, or enters into another inappropriate relationship with someone else.

This involves modelling what a good relationship can look like. I develop this further in Chapter 8, but for here the point is that work on resilience argues that it is never too late to re-establish broken boundaries. As noted by Coleman and Hagel (2007: 13):

> It would appear that even for those who have suffered high levels of adversity at an early age, there are some protective factors that operate in adolescence and early adulthood. ... There is also evidence that, during the adolescent years, involvement with positive peer groups, as well as the impact of a caring and supportive adult, can act to counter early exposure to risk factors (Luthar 2003). One of our favourite articles in the scientific literature on this subjects entitled: 'I met this wife of mine, and things got on a better track' (Ronker et al 2002).

Although we might take with a pinch of salt the prospect of marriage as the answer to all problems, the point here is that a good relationship, even later in life, can be significant in changing patterns of behaviour.

To develop this, it is helpful to look at how risk factors and protective factors can both operate at an individual, familial and environmental level as existing analysis shows that the resilience of the individual, the family or care group and the environment are of equal importance.

Individual, familial and environmental risk and protective factors

The research on risk, resilience and protective factors suggests that the needs of (1) the individual, (2) the family, and (3) the environment must each be considered. Once recognised, they then need to be connected so that a holistic response can position the young person within their relationships, social, environmental and economic context (Rutter 1985, Coleman and Hendry 1999, Newman 2002).

So firstly, risk factors impacting on the individual such as low self-esteem, poor physical and/or mental health and problematic attachments to friends, family or carers have been put forward as affecting sexually exploited children and young people. Research into the young people's trajectories show that low self-esteem, serious drug and alcohol problems, mental health problems, poor school achievement and low perceived control, mean that the young people find it difficult to assert themselves and to form constructive and rewarding interpersonal relationships (Chase and Statham 2004, Harper and Scott 2005). Indeed, as said by Rachael,

> It's only possible to protect yourself if you think you're worth protecting
> (Rachael, aged 17, in Pearce et al 2002: 56)

It is argued that these risk factors might be countered by individual protective factors such as a stronger sense of self-esteem, a positive experience of long-term strong mental and physical health and some secure, good attachments to friends and family/carers.

However, for many sexually exploited children and young people, the impact of negative risk factors outweighs the availability of protective factors. A study of 55 young women showed that 34 of the 55 regularly self-harmed, 26 had been bullied at school, 18 had attempted suicide and all 55 had problems with binge drinking, being drunk at least once a week (Pearce et al 2002). The Barnardo's evaluation of their services showed that of a study of 42 young people (seven young men and 35 young women) that:

> self harm or attempted suicide was identified in 10 cases. The most recurrent issue discussed was the poor self-regard in which young people held themselves.
> (Scott and Skidmore 2006: 29)

Indeed, the young people themselves often refer to this when talking about their experience.

For example, Pat, aged 16 years noted that 'I get into cars with men I don't know, take drugs and do bad things because I am depressed' (Pearce et al 2002: 37). She explored how her feeling of depression linked to her poor self-esteem and how pleased she was when her 'boyfriend' (who abused her physically and sexually and provided her with drugs) gave her attention. It was not until later in the work with Pat that she was able to see how her 'boyfriend' abused her by using her depression and need for reassurance to his own ends. Similarly, Jay, aged 17 years noted that:

> I used to stay in my bedroom for two moths. I couldn't get out. I even tried to commit suicide as well ... I tried to take tablets. I just didn't see point in living no more and because of what my sister was doing to me it kind of, topped it all, and made it worse
> (Jay, aged 17, in Pearce et al 2002: 44)

She was making the connection between her depression, her problems with her family attachments and her behaviour which escalated between intermittent periods of staying in her bedroom on the one hand and running away from home on the other. These individual risk factors make the young person vulnerable to flattery and manipulation by abusive adults.

The traditional grooming model of sexual exploitation: where an adult encourages a young person to become dependent upon them, is based on the adult's ability to exploit the young person's vulnerable mental health. This 'grooming' model has also been applied to the way that particular young people who are looking for friendship are enticed into abusive sexual relationships by paedophiles over the internet (Palmer and Stacey 2004).

As noted, one of the concerns of this grooming model is that it is too firmly based on the premise that the young people are devoid of their own agency or resilience to manage the situation that they find themselves in (Melrose and Barrett 2004). In some cases the young person will be very vulnerable and manipulated to the point that they loose any sense of their own agency, while in others the young person will still be involved in intricate negotiation and man-oeuvring around their developing relationships.

Protective factors impacting on the individual

A strong protective factor for the individual is a more secure sense of self, the confidence in an ability to be self-determined and make decisions for oneself and to be aware of one's own limits of mental and physical stamina to sustain adversity. Some who experience risk factors such as depression, low self-esteem and poor family relationships might be more resilient, more proactive in decision-making and in retaining some control themselves over their situation.

For example, Iona, aged 17 years, had been raped by a boyfriend whom she had left because he was encouraging her to sleep with his friends for money for his drugs. The rape had resulted in a pregnancy and, with social work support, she was able to keep the baby in her own home, sharing child care with her mother. She felt very depressed after the birth of the child and the previous difficulties that she had experienced with her mother re-emerged. They disagreed over the child care to the point that Iona ran from home.

> That's one of the things that made me run away when my son was ten days old. I can't hold him, fine, then you just have him and I'll go about my business. I was on the street for four or five days just eating, Oh God, I can't talk about this … This is just ugh. I used to eat food out of the garbage …
>
> … I ran away for three months, when I couldn't take into more out there. I had no food, no nothing. One thing I believed is, don't ever tell … I got tempted to do prostitution. I've slept in men's houses that I don't know and though every day I ran away. … I used to go out there, I'd sit in a pub, act like, you know I just come work or something, well … I don't have nowhere to go that night …

She explained how she would meet a man who would say:

> ' ... don't worry. You can stay at my place tonight and I will take you to
> your place tomorrow ... ' If he tried to do anything I would go, 'Oh, I'm
> on my period', Why don't you wait till tomorrow, and when tomorrow
> comes I move on. The next man come, I do the same thing. Sleep at his
> place, eat, next morning come out. One day I stole money from one of
> them. I wouldn't lie. I stole £123 and bought myself some clothes and I
> couldn't go back to the same place because that man that I took the money
> from, that's his regular pace so I just decided OK, this is just about it, go
> home. You can't take no more.
>
> (Iona, aged 17, in Pearce et al 2002: 46)

One of the key issues for Iona was her ability to make decisions, to feel in
control of what she did and to be a little self-determined, using her own agency.
Developing the scope to offer sexually exploited children and young people
the opportunity to take some control over their activities is central to the
development of this protective factor. However, as practice shows (Melrose and
Barrett 2004, Scott and Skidmore 2006), this is not simple or without its own
risks. To offer opportunities for young people to express and act on what they
want to active is difficult if it runs the risk of them putting themselves in further
danger.

For example, Tom who was referred to in Chapter 4, really wanted to go
with his boyfriend abroad, where he was promised a 'new start', a happier,
freer lifestyle. Tom saw this as an opportunity to leave his dysfunctional home,
to be in what he thought would be a more supportive environment where his
sexuality would be accepted, and to be with his boyfriend without 'hassle' from
workers. The workers' task was to try to enable Tom to see that the boyfriend,
who was encouraging Tom to sleep with other older men, did not have his best
interests at heart and that although it seemed attractive, the arrangements for
accommodation and ongoing support abroad did not work in his best interests.
Questions ran riot in this situation about the young person's ability to know
what was best for himself, about whether workers should intervene for fear of
being seen as trying to prevent Tom from exploring his sexuality and sexual
orientation and about how to support him in facing up to his family difficulties
rather than run away from them. Sensitive work enabled Tom to continue to
make some decisions for himself about his future training and educational
needs while discouraging him from 'escaping' into the unknown. One of the key
factors in this case was the relationship that Tom was struggling with in his
family grouping. I move now to look at how the family, or the care setting can
play an essential role in creating risk or protective factors.

As noted above, it is proposed that there are three forms of risk factors: (1)
the individual; (2) the family; and (3) the environment. I move now to look at
the second category: familial risk factors such as parental mental and/or physical health problems; patterns of neglect, of physical, sexual or emotional abuse;

criminality within the family; or family histories of being looked after or being in care. These risk factors can mean that resources within the family are stretched and strained, limiting the family's capacity to support the young person. Experience of problems within the family has been identified as a risk factor for young people vulnerable to sexual exploitation. In the study of 55 young women, 53 were regularly running away from home, 47 had experienced physical abuse within the family, and 25 had known experiences of sexual abuse within the home. Thirty-nine of the young women had been taken into care by the local authority (Pearce et al 2002). Only five of the young people from the Barnardo's sample of 42 sexually exploited children and young people were living in 'intact' families with both birth parents. Nineteen of the 42 had spent some part of their childhood in the 'looked after' system, many having experienced a number of changes of carer. Twenty-eight had experienced sexual abuse in childhood, 14 had experienced physical abuse and 20 had experienced emotional abuse (Scott and Skidmore 2006: 17).

These same familial risk factors transcend class and ethnicity divides. The Barnardo's evaluation also goes on to warn against assumptions being made about family background:

> ... service provider perception of a young person's family background and situation was also important – for example, in one case child protection concerns were apparently overlooked because the young woman came from a 'nice middle class family', even though the young woman was deeply unhappy and her parents were violent towards one another
>
> (Scott and Skidmore 2006: 18)

It has been noted that we have very little knowledge of sexual exploitation among young women from different ethnic backgrounds and therefore very little knowledge of whether different groups are affected in significantly different ways to others (Chase and Statham 2004).

However, as explained by Ward and Patel in 2007, the work of a National Society for the Prevention of Cruelty to Children (NSPCC) project for sexually exploited children and young people located in an area with a high Bangladeshi population, showed that their work with sexually exploited Bangladeshi young women identified family conflict and discord amongst some of the families concerned. There were additional pressures placed on these young women who were further silenced by their concern about *izzat* (honour), the impact that their behaviour may have on their family, and its position in the local community. Awareness of this meant that the project workers focused on helping the young person to understand the meaning and implications of izzat to the community while also working with the local projects (such as drug projects and sexual health projects) to make their services more welcoming and accessible to the young women concerned.

The need for services to put time aside for proactive planning on how to ensure they reflect the needs of all young people within their localities has been well documented (Cottew and Oyefeso 2005). This is arising from the concern that some practice interventions have a less interventionist approach with families from minority ethic communities for fear of interfering with cultural values, a fear that has been known to justify a 'hands off' approach (Barn 1993 cited in Lees 2002).

This said, Ward and Patel argue:

> case work with the Bangladeshi young women accessing the project suggested that risk factors could be differentiated into two groups: material risk factors and personal and cultural risk factors. Material risk factors typically included economic and social deprivation, unemployment and household overcrowding. Personal and cultural risk factors included teenage rebellion, education underachievement and family conflict. These though were interlinked. Official data on the borough suggests a significant proportion of the households experience economic hardship and are overcrowded (www.statistics.gov.uk) Indeed, a number of young women presenting to the project indicated they were growing up in households in which poverty, overcrowding and economic stress were pervasive.
>
> (Ward and Patel 2006: 344)

Finally, taking this on board, I want to turn now to look at the environmental risk factors such as poorly resourced housing and local community support provision; inadequate public transport; local safe play and sport facilities; and poor schooling or local employment opportunities that are seen to place undue pressures on individuals and families to cope (Fergusson et al 1994). One of the key environmental factors that have been argued to 'push' many young people into exploitative situations is poverty. The young person's need for money, accommodation, drugs or rewards may, in their eyes, be unobtainable in any other way. They may believe that they are exercising choice, albeit constrained choice, over how to earn their money when few other alternatives are available (Harper and Scott 2005).

For example, something as simple as experiencing a ride in a car, an activity that many might well take completely for granted, is an experience that some young people will put themselves in risky situations to achieve. If the young person has been brought up in local authority residential care, or are part of a family or group home where there is not a car (or the car is old, unattractive or unreliable), they will not have had easy access to the basic status symbol of being in a car. Moreover, the very experience of being in a moving car represents 'going somewhere'.

If this is an experience that the young person has been denied, and they have felt trapped on a local estate or in the radius of one or two streets, the excitement of getting into a car, being seen by friends with a more expensive-looking vehicle, being able to move into another area: a new environment, might override the fear of the risks that they could put themselves in. For example, 'getting into men's cars' has immerged as a key indicator of risk of sexual exploitation (Pearce et al 2002).

In total, 30 of the 55 young women talked of getting into men's cars:

... Nine of the 22 young women from London and 9 of the 23 young women from the northern city who were regularly getting into men's cars were aged between 13 and 15 inclusive

(Pearce et al 2002: 37)

As explained by Sarah, she would:

Go out with my friend. Getting into boy's cars. That's when we used to get the 'beep', 'beep', 'beep' but I never used to know what life was then as well. I used to get into anyone's car, but I never had sex with them or nothing like that. I just went for cruises ...

(Pearce et al 2002: 38)

Not doubting that the individual and familial risk/protective factors are important, I have already questioned whether the focus on the individual and their family constrains discussion to 'child protection' discourses, preventing us from looking at the importance of environmental features such as poverty, geography, and opportunities through education and employment. Raising these questions focuses concern towards the structural and economic circumstances within which the young person has to survive. To raise the significance of the impact of environment on the behaviour of young people prevents interventions from becoming lost within a single approach: one focused only on child protection.

These structural inequalities create their own informal economies which do, by their very nature, both attract and exploit young people (Pitts 1997, Melrose 2002, 2004). However, if we are to take the Every Child Matters agenda seriously, the full range of children's services are to take responsibility for keeping all children safe (DCSF 2008g) and for helping all young people to achieve their full potential (DCSF 2008f). This means integrating the safeguarding agenda within all other interventions aimed at improving services for young people.

As noted, many young people experience a spatial entrapment, leading to some feeling caught into informal economies, with little opportunity to escape from violence. In his work titled 'reluctant gangsters', Pitts (2008) explores this point arising from a study of why and how some young people become involved in gang activities. The social exclusion that can be caused by poverty (i.e. the lack of opportunity to move easily away from one or two local estates, to engage in the commercial world in ways that are portrayed through general advertising, television and film, to access or achieve at school and work) is a key feature for young people who are vulnerable to sexual exploitation (Pitts 1997, Crosby and Barrett 1999, Self 2003).

Familial and environmental protective factors

Work to date suggests that 'joined-up' approaches between housing, leisure and social work intervention can be successful in supporting these young people

(Sheffield 2006, Street Reach 2007). These interventions do appear to enable the young person to achieve independent living if they are supported by a secure relationship with an adult who understands the difficulties facing them and their family or carers. This worker does, themselves, need to be supported in containing the anxiety of managing the problematic circumstances and behaviour.

For example, the Street Reach Project in Doncaster runs a distance learning programme through a partnership agreement between local schools, youth service and the dedicated sexual exploitation project. Young people are invited to create portfolios for Duke of Edinburgh Awards. Being given assistance (an allocated worker, funding to cover travel and regular contact with repeated reminders of the venue and purpose of the meeting) young people are encouraged to attend school-based sessions, youth centre activities and outreach programmes.

The youth worker from the Street Reach Project maintains contact with the sexually exploited young people attending the distance learning programme, helping them to remember the time to meet the education worker, helping them to arrange transport to ensure that they attend, providing follow-up support and encouragement, ensuring that an eye is kept on the peer group dynamics so that one young person cannot prevent another from achieving. With this support, they collect data, drawings, activity charts and personal reviews that contribute to a portfolio of work.

This scheme, although very labour intensive, builds the young person's confidence in working with teaching and training staff, builds their ability to engage and reflect with learning activities and has resulted in many finding part-time employment schemes or jobs within which they can continue their training. The work with the individual young person is linked into the context within which they are placed. Issues arising within their family are referred on to adult services for support. The local peer group dynamics are considered in the group work that develops and the young person, their family and the environment within which they function are incorporated in the design of activities and dissemination of outputs. For example, the project runs award ceremonies where local friends and family witness the young person receiving a certificate of achievement. Such activities not only impact on the individual, but can help to build the confidence of the family and community within which they sit.

The above sections have explored the relationship between risk and resilience and looked at the different important impacts of individual, familial and environmental factors on sexually exploited children and young people. I want to look now at how levels of risk can be assessed to best meet the needs of sexually exploited children and young people.

Sexual exploitation risk assessment (SERA)

The analysis of 55 case studies of sexually exploited young women identified characteristics that distinguished three groupings of young women concerned (Pearce et al 2002).

Category one, low risk, included 19 of the 55 young women. For these young women, protective factors such as a consistent relationship with an identified key worker, access to good preventative work within school such as access to a lunch time club, after school facilities or education social work and contact with other children's services were available and helped to divert them from harm. These young women's behaviour placed them at risk of sexual exploitation, but they were at the early stages of vulnerability and were not yet fully involved in exploitative relationships. They did not talk of swapping or selling sex for favours or reward. The individual risk factors facing these 19 young women were significant, but they still had enough contact with family and community to expect that good protective factors could be built upon.

Category two, medium risk, included a further 15 young women who were either in the initial stages of being groomed for exploitation, being in close attachment with a 'boyfriend', or were talking of swapping sex for accommodation, drugs, alcohol or gifts. These young women were beginning to lose contact with their school and carers. The familial and environmental protective factors that might be able to support them in managing the risks that they were facing were becoming more distant while individual risk factors such as low self-esteem, problem drug and alcohol use were escalating.

Category three, high risk, included young women who self-defined as selling sex. The 21 young women in this category were the most in need, carrying the most problems, including sexual health problems, homelessness, self-abuse and serious drug and alcohol problems. They were regularly running from home and truanting, if not excluded from school. Despite this high level of need, they were the most isolated from any service provision. Few had contact with any members of their family or with past carers and most were unable to make appointments with service providers. They all relied on outreach, or open house drop-in services, to provide them with sexual health advice and with drug harm minimisation programmes.

These were subsequently used in a number of Local Safeguarding Children Boards' protocols to provide a framework around which specific services could be developed. For example, the London Safeguarding Children Board referred to the three categories as:

- Category 1 (low risk): a vulnerable child or young person who is at risk of being targeted and groomed for sexual exploitation.
- Category 2 (medium risk): a child or young person who is targeted for opportunistic abuse through the exchange of sex for drugs, accommodation (overnight stays) and goods, etc. The likelihood of coercion and control is significant.
- Category 3 (high risk): a child or young person whose sexual exploitation is habitual, often self-defined and where coercion/control is implicit.
  (categories taken from Pearce et al 2002 adapted by www.londoncpc.gov. uk/Safeguardingsexuallyexploitedchildren.htm See website for further details including risk assessment and models of intervention)

More recently, following findings from research and practice with boys and young men, and from work with young people sexually exploited through the use of mobile phones and the internet, the following definition of sexual exploitation has been agreed as the central definition for the new Department of Children Schools and Families (DCSF) guidance (DCSF 2009).

The definition followed consultation with the full range of projects, agencies and individuals working with the National Working Group for Sexually Exploited Children and Young People (NWG). A model for the assessment of risk was developed to accompany it. This model is now being used as the assessment framework for interventions with many sexually exploited children and young people.

Debate that took place in developing this framework recognised that the Common Assessment Framework (CAF) used as a basis for assessment of child protection held too high a threshold to be useful for services committed to engaging with the preventative, as well as intensive 'treatment'-based interventions with the individual, the family and the community or local environment.

The SERA model aims to motivate interventions with the young person, their family and local community at both the preventative and the more interventionist levels.

As can be seen, the categories of risk and the SERA risk assessment framework arise from considerable work developed through a range of project experiences. Its adaptation in the DCSF guidance (2009) on safeguarding sexually exploited young people enables both dedicated and generic children's services providers to see where to target their preventative and more interventionist work for sexually exploited young people. I outline below both the definition and risk assessment framework guiding policy and practice within the National Working Group for Sexually Exploited Children and Young People.

The National Working Group for Sexually Exploited Children and Young People (NWG 2008)

Definition of sexual exploitation of children and young people

> Sexual exploitation of children and young people under 18 years involves exploitative situations, contexts and relationships where young people (or a third person or persons) receive 'something' (e.g. food, accommodation, drugs, alcohol, cigarettes, affection, gifts, money) as a result of them performing, and/or another or others performing on them, sexual activities. Child sexual exploitation can occur through use of technology without the child's immediate recognition; for example, the persuasion to post sexual images on the internet/mobile phones with no immediate payment or gain. In all cases, those exploiting the child/young person have power over them by virtue of their age, gender, intellect, physical strength and/or economic or other resources. Violence, coercion and intimidation are common, involvement in exploitative relationships being characterised in the main by

the child's or young person's limited availability of choice resulting from their social/economic and/or emotional vulnerability.

Note: this definition arises from joint work between project members of the NWG.

It is encouraged by the NWG that the risk assessment is used in reference to the following guidelines:

The National Working Group for Sexually Exploited Children and Young People (NWG 2008)

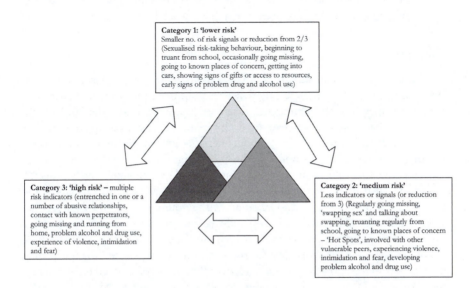

Category 1: 'lower risk'
Smaller no. of risk signals or reduction from 2/3 (Sexualised risk-taking behaviour, beginning to truant from school, occasionally going missing, going to known places of concern, getting into cars, showing signs of gifts or access to resources, early signs of problem drug and alcohol use)

Category 3: 'high risk' – multiple risk indicators (entrenched in one or a number of abusive relationships, contact with known perpetrators, going missing and running from home, problem alcohol and drug use, experience of violence, intimidation and fear)

Category 2: 'medium risk'
Less indicators or signals (or reduction from 3) (Regularly going missing, 'swapping sex' and talking about swapping, truanting regularly from school, going to known places of concern – 'Hot Spots', involved with other vulnerable peers, experiencing violence, intimidation and fear, developing problem alcohol and drug use)

Figure 5.1 Sexual exploitation risk assessment. (The National Working Group for Sexually Exploited Children and Young People (NWG) 2008)

Sexual exploitation: Risk assessment (SERA)

(1) While SERA is to be read alongside CAF it is designed to function independently as an assessment framework for every child at risk of sexual exploitation, whether child protection procedures are deemed to be required in the first instance.

(2) Local Safeguarding Children Boards can incorporate SERA within their protocol for safeguarding sexually exploited children and young people to enable all professionals to be aware of indicators of harm (e.g. Personal, Social, Health and Economic Education, Primary Care Trusts, Looked After Children nurses, Sexual Health Workers, Child and Adolescent Mental Health Services, Youth Offending Teams, Police, Crown Prosecution Service, Drug Action Teams, social workers, residential workers and foster carers).

(3)   Early intervention is essential to prevent escalation of harm. Young people can fluctuate between and within the different categories of the SERA. Movement is not necessarily progressive: that is, a young person deemed to be low-level category one, may suddenly reveal circumstances and behaviours that place them in high-level category three.

(4)   Outreach services (assertive outreach and therapeutic outreach) directed specifically at high-level harm category three have proved to be able to engage and support the young person.

(5)   Exit is possible from either of the stages of risk. Evidence shows that where a Local Safeguarding Children Board has an active protocol, a sub-committee monitoring young people's progress and a dedicated service, young people can be supported away from sexual exploitation.

Conclusion

In summary, it is important to note concerns that have been raised about too strong a focus on risk, particularly if it is seen in isolation from resilience.

For example, a recent conference discussed the impact that the 2012 Olympics would have on sexually exploited children and young people. The debate immediately sprung into thinking about the risks presented: the need for security that can identify paedophiles, the worrying impact of the sex tourism industry and the vulnerability of the young people to an influx of 'strangers'. However, with a different approach, a different 'mind set', the debate could have focused on the resiliencies of some of the young people and projects that work with them. Maybe the impact could be that projects are granted funding for developing outreach services to encourage disaffected and exploited young people to engage with sport. Maybe the potential focus on the Olympics could initiate an interest in team work and in different ways that countries across the world could engage their young people from marginalised and excluded communities.

While the above might well be considered unrealistic, the point is that the dominant perception of sexually exploited children and young people is of them as vulnerable victims who have no other identification but as children at risk. I argue that the danger of this is that it does not include a parallel call for a focus on building the young person's resilience, supporting them and their family or care group in a range of different ways to build their own sense of agency.

In this chapter I have raised these concerns while proposing a definition and a risk assessment model that encourages all agencies, not only child protection services, to engage with preventing and intervening with the problems of sexual exploitation.

6 Doing research in the field of sexual exploitation

If I was a colour I would be orange because I like playing with fire
If I was an animal I would be a lion because they are ferocious and strong
If I could be a famous person I would be Michael Jackson because I like
the way he sings and dances
I like being me because I am funny, kind and happy
(Young woman from Taking Stock, Sheffield, in Sheffield Sexual
Exploitation Service Annual Report 2006–7: 12)

Introduction

In this chapter I want to consider where our knowledge of sexual exploitation comes from and how this determines our understanding of who is affected. I want to explore some of the ethical considerations faced by researchers who are developing research with and on sexually exploited children and young people, questioning whether 'ethically sound' research is able to access the broad spectrum of young people who are most in need. Drawing on a qualitative research study of sexually exploited children and young people I look at both the scope and the limitations of undertaking research in this field.

There are two main questions that are often asked when people enquire into sexual exploitation. 'How many sexually exploited children and young people are there in the UK?' and 'can you give me an example, a profile of a "typical" young person?' These two questions are understandable. There is a desire to know the scale of the problem, to be able to say that a certain number are affected and to have a human face to a story so that the 'general public' understands. This gives people someone that they can connect and empathise with. While the request for data leads to questions about young people's participation in policy debates (questions that are explored later in Chapter 7), the request for a young person's story touches on the practical need for a sound quantitative database on sexual exploitation.

This would be useful for practitioners and researchers as it would give evidence for the need for developments in resources, policy and practice. However, it has not been possible to provide 'numbers' as we do not have a reliable quantitative database in the UK. There are many reasons for this:

Creating a database on sexual exploitation

Although the National Working Group has established an overarching definition of sexual exploitation, safeguarding boards may not have had the opportunity to incorporate this into their practice. They may work to different definitions of sexual exploitation, some perceiving it to be young people involved in prostitution, others seeing it singularly as a form of child sexual abuse (see Chapter 5 for the full definition).

Although it includes this common definition of sexual exploitation, the DCSF guidance (2009) does not advise that data on sexual exploitation be recorded separately by the Local Safeguarding Children Board (LSCB). This means that the type of information available to us will vary between local authorities. Data on sexually exploited children and young people would usually be absorbed into that pertaining to children in need of protection and children with protection plans. As noted in Chapter 2, since the publication of the first government guidance on safeguarding children involved in prostitution (DH 2000), local authorities were *advised* to establish a subcommittee to the LSCB (then the area child protection committee), but were not *required* to monitor data. The redrafted guidance also advises LSCBs to establish a subcommittee on sexual exploitation but again does not set a requirement for the submission of data.

Prior to the original Safeguarding Children Involved in Prostitution (SCIP) guidance (DH 2000), sexually exploited children and young people were recorded through police data under convictions relating to prostitution. This did give us some insight, albeit a limited insight, into the numbers of young people who were visible and identified as 'selling sex' on the street. Data from police cautions and convictions of young people for offences relating to prostitution between 1989 and 1995 show a total of 2,380 cautions and 1,730 convictions for offences relating to prostitution of children under the age of 18 years (Aitchinson and O'Brien 1997).

Information since 2000 would only be available if local safeguarding boards maintained a database of cases of sexually exploited children and young people that they worked with. In the review of the implementation of the 2000 guidance Swann and Balding (2002) noted that 76% of the 111 area child protection committees (ACPCs) in England were aware of children involved in prostitution in their area. A targeted 50 ACPCs (now LSCBs) identified 545 girls and young women and 57 boys and young men involved in prostitution, leading them to conclude that an average of 19 girls and young women and three boys and young men would be abused through prostitution in any given local authority at any one time (Swann and Balding 2002). Harper and Scott reviewed 31 London boroughs in 2004 and found 507 cases where the sexual exploitation of under 18s was identified. Using statistical techniques to estimate the total number of young people thought to be at risk in London at any one time, they predicted an average of 32 per borough and a total of 1,002 in London altogether (Harper and Scott 2005).

As noted, some safeguarding boards do have specialist sexual exploitation subcommittees with associated specialist projects that are equipped to record data of referrals and interventions. For example, Rotherham LSCB refers cases to 'Risky Business': the specialist sexual exploitation project. The Sheffield Safeguarding Children Board sexual exploitation service makes referrals to 'Taking Stock' or SHED (a drug and alcohol service for young people under 19 years of age), both local projects with a service equipped to work with the young people concerned.

Rotherham shows that Risky Business had 118 contacts regarding concerns about sexual exploitation between 2007 and 2008. They received 59 referrals of young people under 18 years of age, delivered a training package to five comprehensive schools and a total of 651 young women took part in preventative work in and outside of school (Rotherham 2008). Sheffield Safeguarding Children Board specialist project noted that between 2005 and 2006 they worked with a total of 56 young people, with 41 new referrals and 15 continuing cases from the last year. The Sheffield LSCB sexual exploitation subcommittee makes a close connection with work taking place for those who go missing. They note that there were missing reports for the 56 referrals, 28% of whom went missing 15 to 20 times (Sheffield 2006: 6).

The Awaken Project in Blackpool showed that they have undertaken 688 joint visits following concerns about sexual exploitation, they had 94 arrests of alleged abusers, with 172 sexual offences-related charges and 31 convictions. Their work showed a 60% reduction in repeat 'going missing from home' episodes and 40% of their total case load was of young people under the age of 14 years (Awaken 2007b). The Safe and Sound Derby Project, a specialist sexual exploitation project for young people in Derbyshire worked with 85 individual cases during 2007–8, ages ranging from 8 to 18 years, including 12 young men and 73 young women. They had contact with 2055 young people for Personal, Social, Health and Economic Education from 1st April to 31st March 2008 and from 1st September to 31st August identified over 2200 in 'risky' situations through outreach (NWG 2008).

Barnardos evaluated 10 of their sexual exploitation services during the two-year period 2003–5. Referred to as:

> the first study in the UK which has attempted to evaluate qualitatively the success of specialist services in achieving positive outcomes for young people who are being sexually exploited ...
>
> (Scott and Skidmore 2006: 3)

data were collected from a sample of 557 young people (Scott and Skidmore 2006: 1). It shows the important insights that can be gained into multi-agency work where information about sexually exploited young people is linked to strategies for children going missing, for outreach detached youth work services and for disrupting and prosecuting abusers.

However, as we do not have an efficient method of tracking how many safeguarding boards actually have subcommittees focusing on sexual exploitation, yet alone an efficient method of recording and collating data from these sub-committees, we have an inadequate, partial UK-wide database. This leaves us without any reliable method of accounting for numbers of sexually exploited young people.

Some safeguarding boards are resistant to establishing a database, recording and accounting system, seeing the demand as an additional burden on already overstretched resources. As noted before in Chapter 2, the enquiries into the circumstances around the tragic case of baby P are raising a number of questions about the distribution of the existing limited resources available for child protection work. There is a fear that if a system for providing data on cases of sexual exploitation were established, a precedent could be set that would open the floodgates to requests for data on other 'specialist interest groups'.

For example, at a training event with members from a safeguarding board which was discussing the establishment of a subcommittee to address sexual exploitation, one of the worries expressed was that it was setting a precedent: a service provision and data recording system that could be argued for by other 'specialist interest groups'. The attendees were fearful that they could be asked for a subcommittee and for data to reveal the connection between child protection and a range of associated problems. For example, they might be asked for data on the relationship between child abuse and problem drug and alcohol use, domestic violence, or gang and knife crime.

Each of these topics could justify a data recording system and a specialist subcommittee to take a lead in planning and developing strategies for working with relevant partner agencies.

The LSCBs were also extremely anxious that with limited resources, they would not be able to resource either the management of a subcommittee focused on sexual exploitation or indeed, manage the influx of referrals that could develop as a result. Discussion followed about the possibility of over-lapping different interest groups so that one subcommittee service the range of different multi-agency interests. However, the fears expressed by the LSCB at this training event are real fears.

There has been an increase in the request for recording, monitoring and accounting within children's services, a request that Cooper and Lousada (2005) have argued might not be so much about needing data as about displaced anxieties (see Chapter 8 for more details). That is, a belief that if the data about the service provision are recorded, they will, by default, be improved. Faced with increasingly time-consuming requests for record keeping, practitioners worry that the time for contact with clients, and for building meaningful relationships is undermined. Data are needed about the numbers of sexually exploited young people in the country and about the sorts of problems and issues that they face. However, the collection of data needs resourcing so that it does not undermine practitioners' scope to engage with the young people concerned.

There are therefore, a number of reasons why we do not have a comprehensive and reliable database that can tell us about the numbers of sexually exploited children and young people in the UK. However, we do have an increasingly informative database of the qualitative experiences of sexually exploited children and young people. As noted in Chapter 5, we have knowledge of the risk factors that both push and pull young people into exploitative situations. We also know of resilience factors that help individuals and their communities to divert from exploitative contexts. However, gathering these data is not without its limitations and problems. I consider these below.

Accessing young people for research: What data do we have and why?

Research carried out through funding from the Joseph Rowntree Foundation on young people and sexual exploitation in 2002 resulted in the proposal that three categories of risk for sexually exploited young people be provided. These were *level one*: young people at risk of sexual exploitation; *level two*: young people engaged in early stages of sexually exploitative relationships and behaviours, talking about 'swapping sex' for favours; and *level three*: young people who were entrenched within exploitative situations and who spoke about selling sex.

Young people did not necessarily move from one level to the other, or remain 'stuck' in one place. As explained in Chapter 5 where the NWG Sexual Exploitation Risk Assessment (SERA) is described, the categories are fluid and dynamic: for example, *level one* being risks facing those who demonstrate the early signs of exploitation, with young people still attached to schools and peer networks; *level two* depicting risks facing young people in the early stages of exploitative relationships, probably beginning to disassociate from education, carers and peers; and *level three* depicting risks facing young people who are entrenched in exploitative relationships, disassociated from cares, professionals and peers (Pearce et al 2002).

Using these levels of risk as a reference point, it is likely that research with young people in levels one and two will be easier to plan and put into action than that with young people in level three. This leads to us holding a better qualitative knowledge base about preventative work and early diversion than about how seriously entrenched exploitation can be understood and managed. Also, more will be known about the young women and white young people than young men and young people from black and minority ethnic groups, reflecting the profile of service delivery and of young people contacted through 'gatekeepers': project workers and service providers. I develop this point further in Chapter 7.

Knowledge of those who sexually exploit young people

A further gap in knowledge is of those who sexually exploit young people. Researching the young people themselves carries risks to the researchers, but arguably less risk than trying to approach the perpetrators of sexual exploitation. The ethical dilemmas related to accessing and interviewing those who sexually abuse young people, meeting ethical requirements around the confidentiality of data collection and the safety of the researcher might well deter researchers from approaching the abusers, unless perhaps through the criminal justice system working with convicted offenders within the prison environment.

Kinnell (2008) and Sanders (2008) have both provided an informative and helpful overview of men and women who purchase sex. Each question the assumption that those who buy sex are necessarily driven by a desire to damage those who sell. However, the focus of this work is on the purchase and sale of sex between adults. There remain gaps in our knowledge about whether all adults are aware of the legal framework that protects young people from sexual exploitation and about the definition of a sex offender that accompanies it. We do not have enough insight into the pressures of local community networks, of gang cultures and of informal economies to understand how some young men or women might act on the knowledge that 'sex sells' and coerce their peers into exploitative situations. More research is needed in this area to help us to understand the reasons some young people and adults are perpetrators of this abuse.

Some important preventative work is being carried out by organisations such as 'Stop it Now' and 'Respect', giving us a stronger understanding of the backgrounds and motives held by potential and actual abusers. Important as it is, this only gives us insight into those who have decided that their behaviour is a problem and are seeking help and support in challenging it.

Undertaking outreach work to engage with those who are actually involved in exploiting children and young people prior to arrest and conviction sets enormous challenges for potential research. One of these is the ethical considerations that need to be addressed. I turn now to look at how these considerations have been incorporated into research on sexually exploited children and young people.

Ethical considerations in research with sexually exploited young people

As suggested, there are a number of important ethical considerations that need to be considered when preparing and undertaking research with sexually exploited young people. Many of the issues facing researchers who are trying to access and research sexually exploited young people are similar to research with other 'hard to reach' groups that have been well documented, the limitations and difficulties being fully discussed (Pain et al 2002, Blake and Butcher 2005).

Although not focusing on sexual exploitation, a particularly interesting debate about questions of access, confidentiality and representation can be found in Ward's assessment of her role in friendship groups of the 'rave' dance culture that she researches. This account gives a helpful insight into some of the ethical considerations in accessing groups who might otherwise appear inaccessible (Ward 2008). Most interestingly, she explores questions about using friends and colleagues as gatekeepers to research subjects, looking at the impact that having to maintain confidentiality can have to these important ongoing relationships inside and outside of the work context.

Risk and research ethics

Some of these ethical issues are addressed by the Economic and Social Research Council (ESRC) which notes the need for full consideration of ethical issues that arise from research involving risk to the researcher and to the researched. These are, in the main, supported by similar statements from the British Society of Criminology (2005), Barnardos and National Society for the Prevention of Cruelty to Children (NSPCC) code of ethics (Barnardos 2008). Ethical procedures have been established so that all social science research within the academy has clear guidance on good practice (ESRC 2006). These ethical procedures encourage researchers to address questions about the risks faced by researchers, the researched and others, such as gatekeepers, who might be involved. The ESRC ethics framework definition of risk encompasses potential harm ' ... both for the research subjects and the researcher ... ' (ESRC 2006: 21) and notes that:

> Risk is often defined by reference to the potential physical or psychological harm, discomfort or stress to human participants that a research project might generate ... as well as the adverse effects of revealing information that relates to illegal, sexual or deviant behaviour
>
> (ESRC 2006: 21)

Researchers are not to be put off from undertaking research that carries risk. Instead, they are to identify what the risks are and how they will be managed. Research is possible with groups that involved more than a minimal risk, such as:

> ... involving vulnerable groups ... sensitive topics ... where permission of a gatekeeper is normally required ... which would induce psychological stress, anxiety or humiliation

If undertaken, such research will require ethical considerations to be fully explored. Barnardos provides a thorough and helpful guideline on how to manage such considerations when planning research, including looking at the researchers' responsibilities towards research participants and issues about the impact of research on young people (Barnardos 2009).

The work of projects undertaking preventative work in schools recognises that a general classroom-based discussion of sexual exploitation or of abusive relationships can be difficult and anxiety provoking for young people concerned. Returning to the three categories of risk, the classroom is likely to contain young people who face risks outlined in category one. Those facing risks identified in categories two and three are unlikely to be in school at all.

For the work to take place in the school, researchers will need to be police checked, will need to know how to engage with the young people in a constructive way and the school will need reassurance that the publication of findings will not place them at risk of being isolated as a problem school attracting 'headline' news. Informed consent will need to be gained from the

child, young person and their parent/carer with a clear statement of how confidentiality will be maintained and how child protection concerns will be followed up. Research that involves young people considering or discussing their
awareness of sexual exploitation will need to ensure that counselling and further ongoing support is available if they are adversely affected by the questions.

Research that aims to explore the impact of sexual exploitation on those
young people who might be categorised as facing risks in levels two and three
carries more complicated ethical considerations.

I will now draw on some of the issues facing myself as a researcher in 2002
when I undertook research funded by the Joseph Rowntree Foundation in
partnership with the NSPCC into sexually exploited children and young people.
This work raised similar questions about ethical issues that have been discussed
elsewhere (Melrose 2002, Coy 2006, 2007).

Research in partnership

This research aimed to look into the choices and opportunities available to
young women who were experiencing sexual exploitation. Although this particular
research was funded to explore issues facing young women, referral routes were
made available for young men who might be contacted during the research.
Future work has aimed at developing research and service delivery with young
men (Palmer 2001, Lillywhite and Skidmore 2007).

It was agreed to focus on young women in the two locations where the
NSPCC provided a dedicated service to sexually exploited children and young
people. One was based in a northern city, the other in an inner London borough.

A process for offering follow-up support to young men who were met during
the course of this research project was instigated. It was developed as an action
research project so that findings could be used to influence practice and policy
development at a local level (i.e. by the dedicated service providers in each
locality) and at a national level (i.e. across the NSPCC and other service
providers).

Young women recruited to the research project were accessed either from
referrals being made to the NSPCC projects or through outreach work, where
research staff, accompanied by NSPCC key workers, went out into the local
streets during the evenings and early morning. Young women were also recruited through snowballing techniques, where those who were in contact with the
research and service provider told friends or acquaintances about the research.

Gatekeepers and research in partnership

The use of gatekeepers to secure access to 'vulnerable' and/or 'hard to reach'
people for research has been reviewed in texts about qualitative research (Silverman 2006). It is widely accepted that the use of gatekeepers benefits research
with 'hard to reach' communities. Gatekeepers can provide researchers with
advice and support about how to contact and engage their 'clients': the research

subjects. They can provide a follow-up service to the researched if the research process has revealed unexplored emotions or practical issues that need service delivery responses. Also, in action research projects the gatekeeper can better apply the research findings to their project development as they will have deeper understanding of its rationale and purpose.

On a more practical level, the partnership arrangements made between the university researchers and the NSPCC meant that safety issues facing both gatekeepers and researchers could be considered together. For example, securing the use of, and insurance cover for, a car that could be used during antisocial hours for outreach work and developing a 'tracking system' that would record researchers' whereabouts through mobile phone contact was established. This meant developing a timetable that would allow a research worker to be accompanied by a project worker on each outreach trip. Through such joint work between researcher and gatekeeper, young people contacted through the research had immediate access to a project worker. This released the researcher to maintain a boundary around their role as information gatherer, rather than 'slipping' into becoming a project worker for the young people contacted.

The early planning of the research considered the potential problem of the involvement of gatekeepers undermining the objectivity of the research, influencing the selection of research subjects and therefore allowing partial view to the problems experienced. However, this was established as a limitation to the research, outweighed by the benefits of having the availability of ongoing specialist support for child protection issues and for a referral point for young people for follow-up if needed.

Boundaries between research and project work

This was extremely important. For example, one evening on the outreach work the researcher and project worker met a young woman, Lorna, aged 17 years. She had just got out of a car where she had been scoring (getting drugs) from a guy. The researcher's notes say that:

> she gave us her number but was intoxicated and not keen to wait around. She had just been bitten on the arm about an hour before we met her – she asked us whether we thought she should go to A and E and get the swelling checked out
>
> (Pearce et al 2002: 81)

Similarly, details of a meeting with Vicki, aged 16, are recorded in the researcher's field notes of an outreach session. She:

> was unwilling to engage further but refused to be taken to a doctor or A and E. She has just been forced to have sex (she would not define it as rape) and was still recovering from her previous abortion. Little was gained for

the contact about education or social work contact other than she says she 'wants to go to college and be a normal girl'

(Pearce et al 2002: 81)

These two situations illustrate the need for a project worker to be available for the young people. Such availability means that the researcher can try to hold onto a slightly detached, more objective position, focusing on the situation faced by the young person while the project worker tries to secure an ongoing relationship that the young person can refer to there and then, or return to at a later date if and when ready.

Both examples also illustrate the need for research with hard to reach and vulnerable young people to be able to 'let go of' the research objectives and focus on the young person's welfare. In neither of these situations would it have felt right for the researcher to pursue questions listed on a semi-structured interview sheet.

As noted with the meeting with Vicki, 'little was gained about education or social work'. Vicki's immediate need for medical attention and therapeutic support outweighed the need for data to be gathered according to a set run of questions. To have asked Vicki to answer questions when she was so distraught would have been unethical. While the researcher ran the risk of losing Vicki as a research subject, Vicki's immediate health needs required a direct response. Indeed, it was the context that she was found in, the situations facing her that became data for the research project, rather than her actual view of her situation at the time. I elaborate on this point further below, referring to the work of Holloway and Jefferson (2000) which explored the context that people find themselves in, and the meanings they give that context as important data for qualitative research.

Confidentiality and child protection

During the early stages of developing the research project, steps were taken to agree a confidentiality policy and child protection procedure. There were concerns that the need to reveal the confidentiality policy to the young people might undermine their willingness to participate with the research. It was recognised that there would also be practical difficulties in enabling the young people to give consent. They might be on the street late at night, under the influence of drugs and/or alcohol and be engaged in violent or abusive relationships with adults at the time.

This would immediately place them as at risk of significant harm. In essence, it meant that all young people contacted for the research would need to be reported to children's services, including the police, as in need of protection. There was a fear that informing the young people that information they gave showing them, or others, to be at risk of significant harm, might put them off from participating. The very target group for research: those who were actively exploited, who might be on the run, dissatisfied with professional services and/ or antagonistic to being supported would be prevented from being involved.

As a result, the research team was able to agree a confidentiality policy that created a higher threshold of 'significant harm' with the local safeguarding children's board. This used the terms 'extreme and immediate danger'. The research protocol noted that if a young person was considered to be in extreme and immediate danger, their information would be shared with the police and the safeguarding children board. This, with a description of the independent nature of the research, was explained to the young women from the outset. As an aside, the interesting thing was that none of the young women we met were worried about their situation being conveyed to service providers. Indeed, although often cynical about the services they had been provided in the past, most wanted support and were keen to be told of an agency that could provide for them.

For example, Sue, aged 17 years, was a regular attendee at the NSPCC project drop-in service. She had been a heroin user from the age of 12 years, and was therefore considered to be a child at risk on the child protection register. She was being looked after by the local authority, but had a history of running from her foster carers and had a number of foster care breakdowns. Sue had participated in the research project and had understood the confidentiality policy and procedure. Sue often appeared at the drop-in centre in distress, with frequent stories of fights with peer groups, of sexual relationships with different adults and with self-abusive behaviour, such as cutting herself. These events and reports were recorded for the purpose of the research whilst the project workers continued to try to support her and updated the safeguarding board on her progress at regular intervals. Unfortunately, there was a fear, and it was a quiet, often unspoken fear, that as with many other 17 year olds, the children's service was failing to provide the intensive support that Sue's circumstances justified because:

- There was no outreach component to the Child and Adolescent Mental Health Services and because supported housing and educational outreach services that could begin to work with the problems did not exist or were inaccessible to her.
- She was approaching 18 years when she would be considered to be an 'adult'.

Although the government has promoted helpful policy initiatives to support young people not in education or employment (NEET) during their transition to adulthood, resourcing constraints mean that the policies do not necessarily translate into practice interventions. All too often young people like Sue are left with little support. Many sexually exploited young people continue to slip through the net and are subject to a waiting game – drifting until they become 18 years when they can be transferred to adult services.

Returning to Sue and the issue of confidentiality, a further example illustrates the need for a strong relationship between researchers and service delivery project workers when undertaking research with very marginalised and damaged young people.

On one occasion Sue arrived at the drop-in centre acting in a very agitated way. She had a number of visible bruises and said that she had just been beaten up by a dealer who was trying to persuade her to work for him, selling drugs to (what he called) her punters. She was frightened that he, and his friends, were following her and were about to attack her again. At the time, there was only the research worker and the project worker available in the drop-in centre.

While the project worker engaged with Sue, trying to calm her and to gather the extent of her physical harm, the researcher phoned the police designated to the project. She noted that Sue and the project staff were in serious and immediate danger. Sue had not wanted this phone call to be made, but the researcher and project worker felt that this was a time when the confidentiality clause needed to be enacted in order to protect both Sue's and the project and research staff's safety. Not only did this incident give an example of the use of the higher threshold of confidentiality but it illustrates how the remit of the researcher can change. The partnership arrangement developed between the NSPCC and the university allowed for this to happen if and when essential. An essential part of managing this and maintaining clear roles and boundaries was in allowing time for joint reflection on the research process and the impact it was having on young people, project workers and researchers.

Safety and informed consent

In the incident above with Sue, it was clear that, as she was an intermittent attendee to the drop-in service, there had been time and occasion to explain the research project to her and to gain her informed consent. The research proposal had to acknowledge the possibility that there might not be the time or occasion to consult the young people fully for informed consent prior to their circumstances being recorded.

For example, the contact with Lorna and Vicki out on the street as described above, meant that their immediate needs had to be attended to rather than time being put aside for a full description of the project with a request for signed consent. In these situations, the project drew on work undertaken by Holloway and Jefferson (2000) that suggests that in some cases, irrespective of the actual stories told, credibility needs to be given to the free associations made within the narrative and to the context within which it occurs.

Returning to the ESRC's view of the need to consult the researched we see that researchers should ensure that the aims and objectives of the project are discussed with research participants in order to secure proper informed consent (ESRC 2006: 21).

However, there are some exceptions as research might need to be:

> ... conducted without participants full and informed consent at the time the study is carried out ...

> (ESRC 2006: 8–9)

In her work researching drug use and drug selling among 'rave' dance participants in London, Ward (2008) looks at some of the practical and ethical issues
involved with the use of semi-covert style of research. She notes concern
expressed by researchers about the ethics of covert research. While recognising
the importance of these concerns, she argues that some activities would never
successfully be studied if covert methods were not employed (Denzins 1968 and
Israel and Hay 2006).

Bearing this in mind, this particular research project with sexually exploited
young people (Pearce et al 2002) noted that the mere fact that a young person was
alone, at night, on the street, under the influence of drugs and in physical pain was
research data in itself. In some exceptional circumstances consent need not be
sought from the young person as their personal details could not be gathered.

Instead, the focus became their immediate welfare needs and a later review of
the context within which the young person had been found. That said, the
gatekeeper and partnership arrangement meant that every young person contacted was given a card telling where and when project staff could be contacted
for follow-up work. While the circumstances of some young women, such as
Vicki and Lorna, might mean that informed consent could not be gained on the
street, there were other situations where even if consent was not given, the
young person should be told that their situation was being recorded and that
information would be passed on.

Research and child protection: The duty to report

For example, there was an occasion where a young woman called Fiona, aged
16 years, met the researcher and project worker at about 1.30 am while she was on
the run from her residential home. She had run because she had fallen out with
some of the other residents and had been targeted by an older man with whom she
had had a relationship. She was very nervous about being identified, and refused
to return home or accompany the project staff back to the drop-in centre.

However, she did understand that her whereabouts would have to be recorded and passed to the police for her own safety. When talking to the researcher,
she agreed that the researcher could record her situation, although was (perhaps
rightfully) very cynical about the possibility of any support services being
directed to meet her needs or those of other young people who ran from home.

She noted that it was the situation that the young people have run from that
needs attention and intervention, rather than (or as well as) the behaviour of
the young person, saying that:

> it was too late now for any help, if services had wanted to help, they
> should have helped in the past
>
> (Pearce et al 2002: 63)

She was aware that if found, she would be returned to a potentially violent
base. She expressed her deep understanding of the ironic position that the mere

fact she was on the run meant that she was in danger and in need, but that she could not access any support services for fear of being retuned to what she saw as a worse situation. There was 'nothing for wanted underage people' because all service providers would have to report her whereabouts.

To have engaged in covert research in this situation might have enabled the researcher to gain further insight into the young woman's feelings and circumstances. However, to have left her unreported as 'missing' would be to undermine her need for safety. It would have left her with the message that being on her own on the streets was acceptable. This was not considered to be an acceptable message to leave her with. She might have been left feeling that some adults were happy to interview her and then leave her unprotected. Her sighting was reported and the residential home was given extra support in working with the peer group dynamics and improving residents' safety. If such research is to be credible, it needs to work within the principles agreed under the safeguarding agenda.

Emotional labour

One aspect of research with hard to reach communities, which is often overlooked, is the emotional welfare of the researcher. This has been explored in full by Melrose (2002) and discussed in Coy's work on her role as researcher and outreach worker with sexually exploited young people (Coy 2006).

Melrose considers the damage that can be done to the researcher, the research process and to the researched if the welfare of the researcher is not taken seriously. Her review of her work with problem drug-using sex workers, addresses the need for the researcher to be able to 'offload' the feelings created by interviewing respondents who express anger and depression. She looks at how hard it is for the researcher to both see, and describe, the circumstances that many drug-using sex workers are faced with. She considers the feelings of the researcher's guilt experienced when walking away, leaving research subjects in situations of unacceptable violence and distress (Melrose 2002).

The preparatory work between the NSPCC and the research team involved securing adequate therapeutic support to staff so that they could sustain the emotional labour associated with the work. Research staff met a therapeutic consultant once a month to discuss the impact that the research was having on them as individuals and on the research process. For example, it was debated as to whether the decision to move from outreach to working with young people who attended the drop-in sessions was motivated by a desire to avoid seeing the dangers and discomforts of young people on the street late at night, or by the desire to engage young people in more project-based activities.

As will be explored further in Chapter 8, working with sexually exploited children and young people can be hard for practitioners to sustain without ongoing supervision and support. The Barnardos statement of ethical research practice recognises, along with other academics working in the field, that it is essential to build non-managerial supervision for researchers into a proposal. If working in partnership with gatekeepers, it is useful, at times, for this supervision to be shared.

Conclusion

This chapter has outlined the key issues to be taken into account when planning or carrying out research with sexually exploited children and young people. It has considered the preparation that needs to take place when developing research projects that might aim to fill gaps in public knowledge and understanding of sexual exploitation. It has addressed the reasons for these gaps and suggested ways that they can be overcome.

It advocates a 'rolling out' of the knowledge and experience to all children's service providers and the general public, not through sensationalist bursts of media reporting that focus on girls in short dresses on street corners, but through a prepared educational strategy that raises public awareness on sexual exploitation.

We need better knowledge for practitioners and the general public about the links between sexual exploitation, violence, gangs, problem drug and alcohol use, mental health and self-esteem, sex, sexuality, sexual orientation and adolescence. This knowledge does exist within existing established projects that are undertaking this work.

If we want to truly advance a preventative agenda we need to establish a fully fledged awareness-raising campaign that takes lessons learnt and knowledge gained out into the public so that:

- Parents and teachers notice the early warning signs and know what to do about it.
- Doctors and health staff in primary care feel part of an information-sharing safeguarding strategy that works in the best interest of the child.
- Law enforcement agencies and those involved in court processes understand how to work with partners to disrupt and gather evidence against the abusers.
- All agencies recognise the support that a young witness will need to withstand the process of taking a case forward against an abuser who they have (in some but not all cases) felt themselves to be in love with.
- Potential and actual perpetrators know that their behaviour is unacceptable and that actions will be taken to prevent and prosecute.

Through supported research work that enables quantitative and qualitative data to be collated and distributed, this may be achieved. Drawing on this information, better early intervention, improved access to targeted and universal provision and stronger disruption and detection of abusers, it will be possible for us to better safeguard young people from sexual exploitation.

7 Young people's participation

'I would get my hopes up about this placement or that placement and then be
told there wasn't the money'

Even if its just a choice between this kid's home or that one, the young person
should still be asked. Even if it's just which bed for the night – this one or
that one?

I might be dead if it wasn't for that project – I definitely wouldn't be sat here
doing this

(Young people from the National Youth Campaign on Sexual Exploitation,
Brown 2006)

Introduction

There are two dominant images of a sexually exploited young person. In both, the
young person is female. Firstly, there is the 'young female prostitute', a media-
dominated stereotype of a young woman hanging over the opening door of a
man's car, on a dark and lonely street. She is either wearing high heels or long, over
the knee, boots. She is always wearing a short skirt. Usually she is white, although
sometimes she is black African/Caribbean. Rarely, if ever, is she Asian. She is
always a 'shadow', an image set against the dim lighting of an urban street.

Then, alternatively, there is the damaged, vulnerable, abused girl in the
corner of a bare room. Again, she is usually white, although sometimes in these
cases, the ethnicity is less transparent. Often there is a door opening, a man
about to step towards her. Invariably there is a tear on her cheek, and, unlike
her counterpart who dares to venture out into the streets on her own, her face
shows fear and dread. These two conflicting stereotypes dominate the public
view of sexually exploited children and young people. The former, the girl on
the street, is designed to lure the reader into the story through the promise of
sex. The latter lures the reader into the story through conjuring fear, sympathy
and outrage at unacceptable abuse.

As with all stereotypes, there are some truths in these representations of
young people's circumstances. Some young women do solicit, some are trapped
in isolated rooms, but these are not the only stories. These dominant images are
limited as they overlook the varied and complex forms of exploitation and

endorse a polarised and restricted understanding of its range and scope. Rarely do newspaper articles address the needs of sexually exploited boys and young men, and when they do address race, it is often with a focus on white girls being abused by 'foreign' men. There are many different circumstances and situations impacting on boys and girls, young men and young women from a range of different ethnic and cultural backgrounds, many of which remain unidentified or under explored.

Some feminists have challenged the dominant gendered discourses that have traditionally focused attention on white young and adult women. Others have challenged the attribution of certain 'places', such as the public domain as 'male' against other places: the private domain as 'female'. For example, some studies have shown differences between black and minority ethnic young people's use of education and social services provisions (Mirza 2007). Others have highlighted how boys can spend time in traditionally 'girls' spaces, such as bedrooms, while girls can spend time in 'boys' spaces such as streets and parks (McRobbie 1991, Skelton and Valentine 1998, Alder and Worrall 2004).

However, little has changed the dominant understanding of gendered informal economies, crime and violence which still appear to create over-simplistic polarisations of the criminal male offender, who operates in the public domain, against the female victim who is trapped within the private domain (Kinnell 2008). This means that some of the complexities and nuances that do take place between men and women, boys and girls in a variety of different settings are overlooked.

In this chapter I want to explore some of these complexities. I look at findings from research and practice to consider how sexual exploitation is gendered. I address how our understanding of exploitation can change when we free ourselves from overarching assumptions that are maintained through binary oppositions that polarise men/boys as perpetrators against women/girls as victims. By breaking away from this limited opposition, we can be more open to awareness of boys and young men being sexually exploited by both men and women.

I also look at work that explores the issues for sexually exploited minority ethnic young people, addressing some of the concerns that have been raised about identifying the needs of young people concerned and about making services accessible to them.

Finally I look at how practice might encourage young people to participate in the development and management of research and in services targeted to meet their needs. I look at some of the different attempts to access voices of sexually exploited young people, considering the problems and achievements of this work.

Gender, boys and sexual exploitation: 'Boys are bad and girls are sad'

As already considered, sexual abuse is understood as 'private', hidden within the home with female victims while offending behaviour is understood as 'public', visible to the general public with male perpetrators (Pitts 2008).

The cross-government Action Plan on Sexual Violence and Abuse notes that while men and boys can be victims of violence and sexual abuse, violence is 'gender based'.

> The over-arching Plan covers all forms of sexual violence and abuse, both recent and historic, and all those affected by these terrible crimes including women, men and children. It recognises the continuum of gender based violence, which represents a major cause and consequence of inequality, particularly for women.
>
> (HMSO 2007)

Understanding violence as gender based places the responsibility for its origins at the doors of patriarchy. ECPAT International discusses this, noting that:

> Sexual exploitation is a manifestation of patriarchy ... CSE is not an isolated practice, but part of a system of discrimination and violence, a socio-economic and political system based on the mercantilism of people.
>
> (ECPAT International 2008: 2)

They argue that when working from this understanding of violence and abuse, preventative work can take place with boys to challenge their potential propensity to violence. They continue by noting that while attention has been targeted to protecting girls from abuse, there has, as a result, been less focus on involving boys and young men as allies to prevent such behaviours. Similarly, there has been less focus on addressing the context within which boys and young men are themselves victims of sexual exploitation and sexual violence (ECPAT 2008: 2).

Some excellent work is being done in this vein within the UK by 'Respect', a non-governmental organisation (NGO) working with young men and running domestic violence perpetrator programmes. Two of their central-identified philosophies are that 'men are responsible for their violence' and that 'men can change' (www.changeweb.org.uk/respect.htm.Page 1).

The impact of poverty on young men

The premise that all violence is intricately linked with patriarchy and gender power relations can be disputed (O'Connell Davidson 2002, Phoenix 2004, Kinnell 2008). Increasingly there have been concerns at an international level about the impact of poverty and war on young men, and the ways that both can encourage and force them into sexually exploitative situations.

A recent article of work carried out in two separate Canadian cities: Saskato and Regina showed that of 40 young men in Saskatchewan involved in the sex trade, 83% started working as teenagers.

> 85% of the young men being aboriginal catering for mostly middle to upper class white men. Sixty-two per cent had some involvement with child-welfare

services and that 78 per cent had a history of running away. Running away often leads young teens to become involved in survival sex, where they trade sexual favours for money in order to pay for food and shelter, experts said. Others turned tricks to pay for a drug habit. McIntyre noted that 75 per cent of those surveyed reported a history of being sexually abused prior to working in the sex trade and 80 per cent had been physically abused. The young men in the study were gay, heterosexual and bisexual

(Kyle 2008: 1)

Both cities have undergone rapid economic growth, outstripping growth in other cities in Canada during 2008 (www.gov.sk.ca). The gaps between those living in poverty and those benefiting from the growth are explored, with the implications for young people surviving through informal economics considered.

Other studies endorse the fact that a range of different boys and young men can be victims of sexual exploitation: that there is no one stereotype. It is not only a gay young man experimenting with his sexual identity who runs the risk of being exploited. Studies show that a range of boys and young men can be accessed through outreach programmes to support them from experiences of sexual exploitation and abuse. In research that took place in three countries: Pakistan, India and Bangladesh, the authors note that the prostitution of boys is not new, but has existed and been manifested in different ways for a long time. The findings of their work show many misconceptions, including that boys selling sex are either homosexual or are part of a sex tourism industry.

Their work suggests that the problem is much:

bigger than previously recognized and that exploiters are local men and in some cases local women

(Masud Ali and Sarkar 2006: 5)

They note that the dominant expectations of masculinity mean that boys and young men can be fearful about revealing their vulnerabilities, hiding the impact of abuse from those who might be able to offer them support. While a range of boys and young men were vulnerable, the study did find some common features amongst those who were exploited, saying that:

age, migration status, experience of sexual abuse and family crisis are some of the most influencing factors which in conjunction with poverty con- stitute greater vulnerability of a boy to sexual exploitation

(Musud Ali and Sarkar 2006: 10)

They note that sexually exploited boys are individuals with diverse and emer- ging sexual identifies. The gay sexual identity that is assumed, and the profile or label of 'rent boy/prostitute' can overshadow the fragile, developing identities. Their practical needs, including their entitlements to support services as sexu- ally exploited boys and children, can also be overlooked.

Boys and young men in the UK

Similar findings are evident within the UK. Lillywhite and Skidmore open their article on sexually exploited boys and young men by saying that:

> 'Boys are not sexually exploited' is unfortunately the view, probably subconsciously, of many of the professionals working with vulnerable young men.
>
> (Lillywhite and Skidmore 2006: 351)

Therefore, the complexities facing child protection practitioners who are working with boys and young men who are clearly victims of abuse can be underexplored and challenging to identify. Similarly, sexually exploited young women who may not conform to the 'victim' stereotype, perhaps because they actively seek sexual relationships in public spaces, can confuse those whose interventions are designed primarily with an image of vulnerable, passive victims in mind.

The lack of visibility of young men's needs has been a common theme arising from research in the area. Davies and Feldman (1992) interviewed 81 young male sex workers in Cardiff and 49 in London, many of whom were under 18 years. This found that pull factors, such as the need for money, were a contributing factor to the reason for selling sex. The income from sex work supplemented low-paid, mundane or, more often, no work at all. The research suggested that sex work was not a central feature to their lives, as many worked spasmodically while maintaining ongoing casual social relationships and relationships with families and carers. Some were offenders, carrying convictions for burglary and car theft, homeless and/or had serious problem drug and alcohol-related problems. This study did question poverty as the one simple causal factor for entry to sex work. Although many of the young men needed extra income, it was evident that other undiagnosed health and emotional problems were contributing factors.

A further study identified specific risk factors that can both push and pull young men into sexually exploitative situations. The Pandora project street work contacts with 87 boys and young men in Bristol over a 12-month period identified 98% as having Class A drugs dependency, almost all had housing problems and 90% had been in care; all were currently, or previously had been, involved in other criminal activities; 20% identifying themselves as heterosexual; and around one-quarter of them disclosed previous sexual abuse (Darch 2004). Importantly, all had experienced crimes against them, from homophobic abuse to rape, and none had reported these to the police.

Lillywhite and Skidmore (2006) note that when young men have been considered in research about sexual exploitation, it has either been under the sexual health agenda, where HIV/AIDs prevention has led to interest in the sexual activities of young men; or through interest in questions of sexual identity and the subculture of the gay community. They argue that while these issues are important, they do not capture the range of concerns that boys and young men bring to the services. They do not necessarily focus on the practical housing, education and social needs of boys and young men who are being sexually exploited.

This point is important, and is something that is reflected in the local UK work that has been undertaken with sexually exploited boys and young men. In 2001, Palmer identified two 'categories' of boys and young men who are at risk of sexual exploitation in the UK. She noted that:

- those 'escaping' from situations where they are vulnerable to violence and abuse, and/or
- those who had experienced familial sexual abuse

were particularly vulnerable to exploitation. The 'missing from home' status could lead them into 'street life', and their experiences of previous abuse could lead them into a 'prostitution life'. She notes that sexually exploited boys and young men have been hidden from services and that unless practitioners, carers, peer groups or parents are actively looking for indicators of exploitation, their needs will remain unaddressed.

Visibility of sexually exploited young men

The question of visibility has been the focus of other studies on sexually exploited boys and young men. Donovan (1991) showed that sexual exchanges between men, and between men and young men, might happen in public toilets, parks, bus/train stations, 'cruising' areas, shopping areas and arcades. This reflects findings from the pilot research carried out for the Association of Chief Police Officers (ACPO) in Nottingham in 1999 (Skidmore 1999). However, these locations are not the only places where the sexual exploitation of boys and young men takes place.

Palmer's work on sexual exploitation and the use of the internet shows that boys and young men are vulnerable to being groomed by both men and women through internet sites and chat rooms (Palmer and Stacey 2004). This has been endorsed by further reviews of abuse over the internet carried out by the Child Exploitation Online Protection (CEOP), explained on their 'thinkuknow' website (CEOP 2008). Lilywhite and Skidmore note that Barnardos young men's project had contact with a number of clients who were sexually exploited via the internet, noting three separate cases: one young man who was stripped, shaved and photographed by a friend of his so-called older 'boyfriend'; a 15 year old who was groomed over the internet by a man in his 30s; and a young man whose photograph was placed on a website where men sell sex (Lillywhite and Skidmore 2006).

Despite some projects developing focused and targeted work with young men and despite the National Working Group for Sexually Exploited Children and Young People (NWG) developing, with Safe and Sound Derby, a national forum for work with sexually exploited boys and young men (Young Men's Forum, NWG 2008) there has been little research into the situations facing sexually exploited boys and young men.

Themes from research about sexually exploited young men

From the work that has taken place, there are some reoccurring themes. One is that because of the pressures to conform to gendered stereotypes, boys and young men might feel that they cannot, or should not disclose the fact that they are victims of sexual exploitation. Similarly, practitioners and researchers may not be thinking about boys' needs or looking for them as recipients of their services.

Another is that boys and young men are affected by similar risk factors for sexual exploitation as girls and young women, being vulnerable to grooming, to the need for money to support drug and alcohol problems, needing somewhere to sleep when running or missing from home and often having experienced a history of abuse and neglect. Apart from being mindful of the locations where exploitation takes place and the power dynamics involved, the basic premise of good child protection work and good youth work applies for interventions with young men as well as with young women. There is no 'secret' remedy to a good service for young men. A good service can be developed alongside the provision with young women. Both male and female practitioners and young people might need their own space to develop and deliver the service, but the essential ingredients to good child protection work is applicable across the gender divide.

Finally, boys are not necessarily young gay men experimenting with their sexuality. However those who are should be given the right and freedom to experiment within safe, age-appropriate boundaries.

The lesson for our developing work with young men is that if we neglect these complexities and overlook the needs of sexually exploited young men, we undermine the rights of all young men to equal access to service delivery and we fail to challenge the gendered stereotypes that prevail within media and public perception.

Minority ethnic young people

The dominant image of a sexually exploited child or young person is of them as a white young woman. This has a negative impact on the extent and quality of service provision to black and minority ethnic communities.

The recent focus on trafficking as a social problem has led to a polarised image of the sexually exploited black or minority ethnic young person being from abroad. This can run the risk of polarising a black young person as an outside 'other' against the white young person as an 'inside' UK white young person. The recent legislation and guidance from the UK government is that once identified as trafficked, a young person from abroad should be safeguarded in the same way as a UK national, with the right to remain in the country until they are 18 years

(DCSF 2008e). Putting the issue of trafficked young people to one side for a moment, it is clear from research that it is not only white young people who are sexually exploited in the UK, but that the risk factors of poverty, disadvantage and abuse exist within all communities (Ward and Patel 2007).

The limited evidence that we do have from research shows that black and minority ethnic young people experience sexual exploitation, but that access to children's services support varies for different racial and ethnic groups. For example, the data of black and minority ethnic young people's reception into care shows that while black African and Caribbean young people are disproportionately over-represented in the 'in care' population, Asian young people are not (Coleman and Brooks 2009).

When information about the children and young people going through safeguarding children's boards for sexual exploitation is recorded; if the racial and ethnic origin of the young people concerned is noted; and if this could then be compared to the population as a whole within the locality, we would be able to begin an analysis of the extent of sexual exploitation between communities. We could consider the impact of racial and ethnic origin on referral processes and availability of services. Some local authorities have kept records of the ethnicity of children being safeguarded against sexual exploitation.

What is known about the ethnic origin of sexually exploited children and young people?

A breakdown of data of 47 new referrals to the Sheffield Sexual Exploitation Service in 2006 to 2007 showed that while 77% of the referrals were white British, 2% were white Irish, 4% were black British Caribbean, 4% mixed white and black British Caribbean, while 2% were other unnamed ethnic groups and 11% were unknown (Sheffield 2007). Data from the Awaken Project in Blackpool similarly show referrals from black and minority ethnic communities (Awaken 2007).

Other data come from research work undertaken through NGO services. The Barnardos evaluation of services in 2006 noted that of a qualitative sample of 42 young people (35 young women and seven young men), 69% were white, 7% black, 5% Asian and 11% dual heritage (Scott and Skidmore 2006: 16). Research with 55 young women from two different localities, one inner London borough and one northern English town, involved 38 young women who self-defined as white British, 3 who self-defined as Black African/Caribbean, 3 mixed-race white British and black African Caribbean, 2 Bengali, 5 Bangladeshi, 2 defining as Somali, and 1 as mixed-race Maltese and Turkish (Pearce et al 2002: 30).

The Barnardos young men's project also works with young people from minority ethic backgrounds, with roughly half of their clients being black or of minority ethnic descent. This, as noted by Lillywhite and Skidmore (2006), reflects the demographic composition of the area within which the project is placed. They note that once a young man has been referred to the project, race is rarely a block in his engagement with staff.

This work suggests that while sexual exploitation can be a problem within all communities, not all young people affected might be aware of the services available to them or feel able to approach service providers. Added to this, the service delivery may not be designed with black and minority ethnic young people's needs in mind (Ward and Patel 2007).

Multiculturalism and service provision for sexually exploited young people

There is little research that has been specifically targeted towards considering why those experiencing sexual exploitation in different local communities may be denied access to the services that could help them. Ward and Patel consider this, noting the need to engage in a retrospective analysis as to why a cultural blindness may exist. They note that the policy agenda of multiculturalism has been criticised for 'its failure to recognise issues of power and conflict within minority ethnic communities ... and the reluctance to intervene within family and community' (Ward and Patel 2006: 349).

If a cultural blindness follows the dominant theme of multiculturalism within the UK, service providers and practitioners are discouraged from thinking beyond a generic provision for all. The critique of the multicultural approach is that it negates the impact of racism, allowing blame to fall on those who do not feel able to access the universal services rather than resting responsibility on those providers themselves to identify need and adapt their service (Mirza 2007).

Without an active policy that targets minority ethnic and black young people, most services, research and evaluations of practice will reflect the issues raised by those who do access the services: which is, in the main, white young people. As explored in Chapter 6, there are many important ethical considerations that need to be accounted for when undertaking research with sexually exploited young people. Gaining access to them through 'gatekeepers' is one way to ensure that the young people participating in the research are supported, as the questions and activities that focus on their behaviour and circumstances could raise unresolved and painful issues. This means that researchers will, by default, be limited to access those the gatekeepers are working with at the time. Although gatekeepers and researchers could work together to improve access to targeted communities, the service providers also need to feel confident that they can maintain a service delivery for the young people once contacted.

There is still little work undertaken to explore how race, racism and cultural diversity impacts on the issues presented by sexually exploited young people in the UK. Ward and Patel (2007) addressed some of the considerations for young women and their workers in a National Society for the Prevention of Cruelty to Children (NSPCC) project in London. The referrals to the project reflected the demography of its location where 30.5% of the population were Bangladeshi, 2.1% Indian, 1% Pakistani, 1% other Asian and

44.2% are white British (GLA 2007). They note that 50% of the case load between August 2003 and 2004 were young women of Bangladeshi origin, 23% were black Caribbean, black African, Turkish and Maltese, and 16% were white British. The project had been developed in the borough through close cooperation with local service providers and employed staff that represented the ethnicity of the locality. This was important in enabling the young women to feel comfortable about accessing the service, feeling that the workers would understand and be sensitive to their needs.

However, it is important to note that the engagement of black and minority ethnic young people with specialist sexual exploitation projects should not depend only upon the appointment of black and minority ethnic staff. While this is helpful, it is not an excuse for projects with all white staff to fail to address the need to make their services accessible to the full range of young people within their locality.

The impact of risk factors on black and minority ethnic young people

The issues raised by this work with Bangladeshi young women in London included questions about risk factors, economic conditions and familial cultural pressures.

Ward and Patel note that the:

> main risk factors deduced from the case load work with the Bangladeshi young women could be delineated by material risk factors, such as economic and social deprivation, unemployment and household overcrowding, and personal and cultural risk factors such as teenage rebellion, educational underachievement and family conflict. These though were interlinked
>
> (Ward and Patel 2007: x)

The London borough in which the sexual exploitation project was located has a significant proportion of households who experience economic hardship and are overcrowded. A number of young women report to be growing up in households in which:

> poverty, overcrowding and economic stress were the pervasive conditions in which they lived
>
> (Ward and Patel 2007: x)

This, often combined with familial abuse and disruption, means that the young women went missing from home.

The running away from home, and the risks of sexual exploitation that this carries, is a familiar problem for those working with sexually exploited young people. The additional difficulty faced by some of the Asian young women was in managing the extent of disapproval they would meet from their local community on return from running away. Although, of course, not all families were unsupportive or disapproving, many young people were fearful for their physical and emotional wellbeing, and worried that they would be punished for acting against the expectations of their community.

Izzidien (2008) explores this further in her study of Asian children's, young people's and women's experiences of domestic abuse. She found that although there were few differences in the levels of abuse between Asian and white women and children, the way that it was perceived and experienced by south Asian women was different. The powerful impact of *izzat* (honour) and *sharam* (shame) within the community could make women and young people fearful of incurring the wrath of the extended family. This meant that they may not disclose or highlight abuse. Ward and Patel continue with this theme to argue that:

> Because of the sexual modesty of much of the Bangladeshi community, the sexual relationships being engaged in were forbidden, and for this reason were usually secret and highly hidden
>
> (Ward and Patel 2007: x)

The impact of izzat and sharam on Asian young and adult women is explored further by Meetoo and Mirza (2007) who note the extent of the concern which involves threats as serious as murder being hidden under the banner of 'honour killings'.

Ward and Patel's work did note anxiety amongst practitioners who struggled with concern that Asian young women may be at risk of sexual exploitation, but that they were not delivering a service for them. Indeed, this anxiety could become compounded by a fear of upsetting the young women's modesty by suggesting that they might be in sexual relationships, a modesty that is expected more of Asian young women than their white counterparts. Ward and Patel noted that when a practitioner did refer a young woman to the sexual exploitation project, it was at a point in time when there was a lower threshold of risk than might be the case for the young women's white counterparts. That is, the referrers may be more anxious about sexual activity of a young woman from Asian origin.

This raises a complexity in some of the findings of the research into children's services interventions with black and minority ethnic families. Concern has been expressed that children's services have, in contrast, a less interventionist approach, either leaving families to care for themselves or feeling afraid that an intervention might appear as 'racist' (Barn 1993, Barn et al 2005).

What is evident from this research is that much more needs to be done to encourage practitioners, policy makers and researchers to address the impact that race, racism and cultural diversity may have on the experience of and provision for sexually exploited young people. One start towards working on this is to create a stronger forum within policy, practice and research for the voices of young people themselves.

Young people's participation: Young people's voices

There has been a rapid development of awareness of the importance in encouraging young people to participate in the governance and policy development of the services designed to meet their needs. This has included services for sexually exploited children and young people (COE 2007).

I want to look now at some of the lessons that can be learnt by engaging young people at two levels. Firstly, at engaging them in activities where their voices can be heard by the 'general public'. In this way, they have the opportunity to 'tell their story' and to identify the range and diversity of issues they face. Secondly, I want to look at engaging young people in the governance of project service delivery and in research.

Young people's voices: Different stories

Reflecting on my previous experience as a youth worker, some of my most significant conversations with young people were either when we were in a minibus, travelling to or from the project or going out on a trip; or whilst doing an activity, such as photography or cooking in a kitchen. Sometimes good conversations about difficult topics came at the most 'random' moment, perhaps when just happening to be at a sink, a mirror or at the point of locking up the building.

As noted in Chapter 8, the moment the young person chooses to talk needs to be grabbed as an opportunity. It is more likely that this opportunity would reveal better insight into the young person's feelings than those revealed in a fixed appointment at a time chosen by the practitioner. Young people are unlikely to attend a fixed 'therapy' session each week or to 'spill the beans' in the early stage of a relationship with a key worker.

Engaging with the young person takes time and means working at developing a relationship with them. The premise to 'relationship-based thinking' as explained by Howe (1998), is that practitioners need to be flexible, using the opportunities that arise, wherever they may be.

Young people's participation: Building trusting relationships

A number of specialist sexual exploitation projects use a range of activities developed through flexible youth service approaches to engage young people in 'project work' that helps them to build trusting relationships. Each of the three larger children's charities (Barnardos, NSPCC, the Children's Society) have a range of activity-based games, toolkits and work tasks that are easily accessible on their websites that can be used to this end. Other smaller projects run similar activities. For example, the Annual Report 2006–7 from Street Reach in Doncaster (www.streetreach.org.uk) notes that:

> our priority therefore is to build an early relationship or trust with the young people which enables us to maintain regular contact. During this

time we can offer and deliver a wide range of activities and support that is flexible enough to cater for each young person's individual circumstances

(Street Reach 2007: 15)

There are some key words here: relationship, trust, regular contact, range of activities, flexible support, individual circumstances. Although there is no one stereotype of the sexually exploited young person, there are some common features to engagement and delivery of an effective service, captured above in the identification of the need for a trusting relationship.

Meeting with the young people each week, projects can maintain contact with sexually exploited young people who might not be attending school, but who are motivated to engage in educational project work. In Doncaster, a distance learning programme works by the young person building a portfolio of work, recording activities undertaken at each meeting with project staff, including submitting their drawings, collages from magazine cut outs, photographs of outings and their writing of stories, poems. Through engaging with such activities, the young people not only have the opportunity to explain their own position through their art work, their drama activities and their writing, but they also gain accreditation, a certificate of achievement that they can take with them into the future.

Young people's involvement in creative work

Another example of similar activities that enable sexually exploited children and young people to express their views is shown through a music project run by the Safe and Sound Derby Project. The following song lyrics were written by a young woman from the project, and with her permission, was published in their annual report (Safe and Sound Derby 2008). The song has been played at a number of events, including the national 'Safe and Sound Derby' and NWG conference.

Not only does it portray a 'message' through the lyrics, but it challenges the idea that a sexually exploited young person cannot be creative, cannot produce a high-quality outcome and take responsibility for its use as an educational tool.

Out late at night, cant you see this ain't right
Why are you doing this? cant you see you put yourself at risk?
Always out late, drinking and taking drugs with your mates
You've let yourself into the vulnerability gates
You hear about kids never seen again
Picked up and exploited by women and men
They give you things then they give you a ring
It sounds so good you'd do anything
Being exploited and have no money
At first it was ok but now it ain't funny
Your all alone, you'd rather be safe at home

Your scared, you wonder if anyone cares
They've took everything, even your bling
You are scared and you can't pretend
There's only one way that this is gonna end.

The music project was run by a trained and supported Safe and Sound Derby project volunteer, a graduate from a local university. He ran a music workshop activity where an interested young person was given a one-hour slot to work with him on music activities. The young person would also be given an additional one-hour slot with their project worker.

It was not expected that the young person would just 'turn up' to the activity. Complicated arrangements had to be in place to arrange for either a taxi to collect the young person from their home and bring them to the project, or for a project worker to collect them. The activities at Safe and Sound Derby are usually provided to secure a one-to-one relationship between project worker and young person. Some group-work projects are run, but these need careful planning. The selection of which children and young people work together needs approval through the safeguarding process, to make sure that the dynamics between the young people are safe and contained.

The engagement of the individual young person with the activity comes after the project worker has built a relationship with the young person. Each young person signs a confidentiality form prior to the work taking place so that they know that confidentiality will be maintained unless they disclose that they, or another they are in contact with, is in significant harm or engaged in criminal activities. The reality is that many of the young people worked with will be involved in such activities. However, the confidentiality form ensures that they know that they, or others involved, must be provided with support and follow-up services to meet the needs they identify.

The project recognises that as every young person is different, it is helpful to have a range of different activities available to choose from. The point is that if the young person can do something that they enjoy, it is this enjoyment and sense of fulfilment that is important. The outcomes were relevant, but it was the process – a process that evolved enabling the young person to have some fun and to enjoy their activity for a while – that was the key. The young woman who wrote and sung the song quoted above, engaged with the music project as she enjoyed listening to music and was motivated to write lyrics about herself.

She started writing about herself and what was happening to her in her life. As the work progressed, she started to become more reflective about what was happening to her. After three or four months she wanted to record the music, having something she could take away with her. The local city council gave the project access to their recording studio for two hours for free and the young woman worked with the project worker and other technicians to record the song.

As a result, the young woman was able to take some control in changing her circumstances and eventually it was felt that, apart from the occasional 'catch up visit', she could be taken off the ongoing list of young people in need of supported case work.

The young woman's motivation for writing and singing the song was also, in part, to try to stop other young people getting into the problems that she had experienced. This desire to communicate what has happened and to feel that efforts can be made to stop others going through similar pain is a useful stage in recovery: it is an important step in the young person's ability to step back, express emotion and engage with others.

There are a number of excellent examples of similar project work with young people from the small number of dedicated projects working directly with sexually exploited young people across the country. Some result from interventions that are more structured, some supporting young people who need less focused support, who might be able to take a more measured, and considered approach to their situation.

Examples of activities used to engage young people

Picklington and Lothian (2007) have produced a helpful work book titled 'Friend or foe?' to be used as part of the sexual exploitation and relationships education programme in Sheffield. This work book takes young people through a number of scenarios to consider by enabling the reader to follow some young people's diary entries, posing questions at different stages to encourage discussion. It has been used as a preventative tool in sex and relationship education as well as being used with young people who are sexually exploited, the scenarios showing them that they are not alone and that other young people have struggled with similar problems.

For example, one scenario notes Liam, aged 15 years, becoming increasingly frustrated by his parents' concern with his developing relationship with a peer, James. Liam's parents see James as a bad influence. However, as James introduces Liam to Nick, an older man who provides CDs for the boys to sell, we see Liam's parents being influenced by Nick, believing him to be a good influence as he appears to be encouraging Liam to attend school more often. Liam then becomes more dependent on Nick and finds himself owing money and having to repay him by 'being' with older men. The scenario cleverly opens the opportunity for young people to look at potential problems with coercion, peer group dependency, parenting, school attendance and financial independence.

Examples of activities such as these all work on the premise that young people may not be ready to engage in traditional therapeutic methods to address their problems but may take part in activity-led events that will both help them to express their feelings and build their confidence in their ability to produce an outcome. Involving the young people in this way through the use of trained and experienced staff can help young people to develop a voice, telling their different stories of how sexual exploitation impacts upon them. With their permission and encouragement, these stories can be used to help other young people and adults to understand some of the complexities involved in different forms of exploitation.

Pearce's work with projects in Northern England and London (Pearce et al 2002) involved young people telling their stories through interviews with researchers as well as through project activity work. One 14-year-old young woman who had a serious problem with heroin misuse was referred to the project as she was being 'groomed' into an abusive relationship by an older man she called her 'boyfriend'. The poem that she wrote has been widely used, with her permission, at conference presentations to illustrate the depth of her understanding of the issues she was facing.

She believed she was addicted to heroin, something that she knew was not doing her any good; she knew that having sex with other men was 'robbing wives'; she knew that she was suffering from a depression that pulled her down and that she was experiencing sudden and strong mood swings. She would attend the drop-in service when running from school or home, or when distressed by her circumstances.

There was no regular pattern to her attendance but by maintaining an open door policy and by supporting her to express what was happening to her, the project worker had been able to develop a relationship with her. She was not ready for direct therapeutic work or for engagement in dialogue that made her feel bad about what she was doing. She ran away from this sort of intervention. What she was able to do was to engage in an activity that gave her the chance to tell her story and to express her feelings about what was happening to her.

Heroin by Fi, aged 14

Feel the pain, feel the strain, feel the swelling of the brain.
Sitting down, walking round, wishing you were underground.
Knowing me, knowing you, wishing no one ever knew.
Drugs, shrugs and funny looks, cooking up, throwing up, giving up,
    cleaning up.
Laying down, coming down, feeling like a stupid clown.
Cold turkey, robbing an old lady. Little baby, big girl, bad girl, little girl,
    stupid girl.
No regrets, lots of debts, taking lots of stupid tests.
Hurting lives, robbing wives, wondering why you should not die.
Feeling sorry, feeling low, feeling like you want a blow.
Locked up, knocked up, blocked up, cooked up.
Falling down, feeling down, looking around, spinning round,
feeling like you're not worth a pound.
Wrong crowd, no longer proud, knowing this is not allowed.
Higher than a cloud, lower than the mud, never really thought about giving up.
Living dead in the red gouache, anywhere except for bed.
Walking, waiting, anticipating, never knew that you were breaking.
Want to go, want to stay, don't know what today.

Involving young people in research

In this research project, activity-based work with young people was seen as a method of gaining access to their stories. The focus of debate on young people's involvement in research has been to encourage researchers to consider young people's views in the development of the research questions, design, analysis and dissemination of the findings. This follows the tradition of young people's participation – working not as research 'for' or 'with' but towards building research 'by' young people. A network has been established to encourage this focus (Children and Young People's Participation Learning network www.uwe. ac.uk/solar/childparticipationnetwork/home.htm) and academics are increasingly debating how this approach can be a positive development to research.

Murray (2005) looked at the involvement of children and young people in research in the field of adoption and fostering in the UK. Based on a review of 182 research studies, she noted that 53% involved children and young people in the process of developing and running the research. She looked at why children and young people were involved, how the 'gatekeepers' managed the process and the way that researchers supported young people's participation. Interestingly, although the ethical dilemmas involved in engaging young people were expected to be the main consideration of the research projects, the role of the gatekeepers became the focus for concern. Many gatekeepers were felt to be 'protecting' themselves and their projects from being exposed, using the need to safeguard the child as a means of safeguarding themselves from view. It was questioned whether the gatekeepers were protecting children and young people from the harm that could be caused by participating in an activity, or whether they were protecting themselves from losing control over the young person's case work.

Reasons for young people's participation

This leads to one of the main considerations in the debate about young people's participation. Do practitioners, policy makers and researchers really want young people to have a role in developing the service or research proposal, or may this create challenges that we are not ready, or not equipped to deal with? Is the participation agenda driven by a need to be seen to be doing the right thing – responding to a trend of involving young people in governance issues, or is it driven by a genuine conviction that young people benefit from involvement and that their participation will be useful to them as individuals and improve services for others?

Hart (1997) addressed these questions when he designed his 'Ladder of participation'. At the bottom of the ladder we see a situation where young people are manipulated. There is a token gesture to involve them with decision-making but their views are not taken seriously and they are manipulated to support the dominant adult/practitioner voice. The next step shows the young people to be seen as decoration. They are invited to meetings or conferences so that it looks as though participation is taking place, but they are patronised, rather than taken seriously. We then climb further up the ladder as young people are involved more constructively as equals in participation, with genuine efforts to inform them about the structures and processes involved, starting to consult them properly about the questions and agendas being approached. This, however is still not true participation as the young people are contributing to the adult/practitioner agendas. The full participation comes at the top two rungs of the ladder as the young people are able to take a lead and initiate action, with a genuine sharing in decision-making being achieved (Hart 1997).

I see this represented in a see-saw: with a balanced initiative between identifying the adults' agenda (in a manner that can be fully understood by the young people involved), and identifying the young people's agenda. Through this balancing, a participatory model can be developed. If the onus is either disproportionately on the adults' or young people's side, the power balance will tip either way and participation will not be achievable (see Figure 7.1).

It is noted that participation comes alongside support. This addresses the very difficult and often unspoken issues around power dynamics between young people and adults, dynamics that are particularly pertinent when the young person concerned is damaged, angry, disturbed and/or abused by adults in the past.

The very real question returns about who should participate, when and why. The Council of Europe Convention on Safeguarding Sexually Exploited and Sexually Abused Children and Young People (COE 2007) notes in Chapter 2, Article 9: that:

> each party shall encourage the participation of children, according to their evolving capacity

The important focus here is on the young person's evolving capacity. A young person in crisis and in need of immediate support and protection should not be distracted into expectations of governance participation.

The UK National Plan 2001 'Safeguarding children involved in commercial sexual exploitation' (DH 2001) noted that consulting sexually exploited children and young people was to be an aim of all local authorities in developing their services. One initiative that aimed to do just that has given some important and helpful lessons to take into future initiatives in this area.

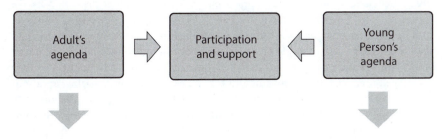

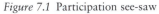

Figure 7.1 Participation see-saw

Brown (2006) explores the work of the National Youth Campaign on Sexual Exploitation which was a joint initiative between the Children's Society and ECPAT UK. The initiative for this came from two reports. A participative research with women and young people with experience of prostitution was commissioned by the Home Office in 2002. This cites 'studies which note that exposing vulnerable young people to political lobbying and media can be problematic as the potential for distorted reporting can cause additional distress for the young person concerned' (Taylor Brown HO 2002: 2). The other, 'More than one chance! Young people in prostitution speak out' highlighted the importance of consulting young people in the development of provision targeted to meet their needs.

In her review of the National Youth Campaign, Brown noted that the Safeguarding Children Involved in Prostitution guidance (DH 2000) supports the Children Act 1989 by restating that the young person's 'wishes and feelings are ascertained and taken account of' (DH 2000: 31) and that 'the child is an important contributor in addressing these issues' (DH 2000: 21).

She identified the fact that current policy and practice has been developed by adults with little, of any consultation with young people and that young people were often perceived as too vulnerable or chaotic to be involved in decision-making (Brown 2006).

Brown notes that young men and black and minority ethnic young people were under-represented in the campaign; of 126 young people who took part, 12% were young men and 11% were black and minority ethnic. She identified that, as confirmed in research and practice, many young people don't see themselves as exploited. This meant that their involvement with a participation project for sexually exploited young people was problematic for them, as they might not want to identify with the main title, or theme of the work. Despite this, the campaign engaged with a range of young people, produced a newsletter, contributed to an exhibition of their work, contributed to the government consultation on the prostitution strategy (Paying the Price 2006) and ran a workshop at a national conference.

Conclusion

In this chapter I have argued that young people's voices, feelings and opinions are best accessed through youth work techniques that allow spontaneous engagement and respond to the opportunities for engagement presented by the young person. This means dedicated services having the flexibility, resources and staff support systems to facilitate relationship-based interventions. I have also noted that young people can play an important role in guiding the development of research and service delivery, but that this must be child or young person centered. It must be meaningful for the young person, creating situations where they understand the role being asked of them and can see responses to their suggestions made. I move now, in the following chapter, to look at some of the therapeutic needs that arise from such activities with young people, considering the support that is needed for staff in carrying out this work.

8   Therapeutic outreach

young people arrive at Barnardos' services with multiple difficulties, with a long history of problems in their family and in school. Most have lives blighted by substance misuse, abuse and exploitative relationships. Such vulnerable young people need a long term commitment from skilled staff working within a supportive environment with a positive policy framework and a secure funding base

(Narey 2006: vi)

Introduction

This extract from Barnardos' Chief Executive highlights the need for long-term interventions from trained staff working within a supportive environment to meet the many needs presented by young people who use their services. All too often poorly supported residential care workers, teachers, youth workers and volunteers are faced with very complex cases of sexually exploited young people, and have little, if no, access to training to help them to understand the issues involved. Services often rely on temporary staff employed on short-term contracts. These staff can be responsible for generating their own income on a year-by-year basis.

This is not an acceptable foundation for a service that is trying to establish and maintain therapeutic relationships with young people who have experienced a range of placement and relationship breakdowns. They might have a number of physical, sexual, mental and emotional health problems; repeatedly go missing; and feel disassociated from school and peers. In light of all of the work undertaken by the Department of Children Schools and Families (DCSF) and other central government departments in securing a constructive policy framework for sexual exploitation, local provision from both voluntary and statutory sectors must be resourced to provide an appropriate service to sexually exploited children and young people.

In this chapter I want to focus on Narey's call for recognition of the problems carried by individual young people and for the need for trained and supported staff (Narey 2006). I will look at some of the lessons that can be leant from therapeutic interventions with young people, addressing the importance of considering the dynamics that can occur between the individual practitioner and young person in the development and delivery of a service.

The individual and their social and economic environment

In earlier chapters I have argued that service responses which focus only on the individual sexually exploited young person and their family run the risk of isolating the individual young person as the problem. Rather than their social and environmental circumstances being considered, the young person's and their family's behaviour, their personal histories and capacities to manage difficulty become the centre of attention. While the focus is on the young person and their family, the poverty, the social exclusion and disadvantage they experience can be ignored. The damaging and detrimental impact of the environment is not addressed, and the practitioner is left on their own, held responsible for improving the young person's behaviour. Instead of the young person and their family being understood as a part of the economic and environmental context that they inhabit, the practitioner is set the unfair challenge of changing the individual without redress to, what is often seen to be, the genesis of the problem.

What I do want to highlight here is that although I am looking at some of the lessons that can be learnt from good, supported therapeutic interventions, I am not advocating that these will be useful if seen in isolation from other forms of support. They are one important part of a range of interventions that need to take place at the individual, family/care group and community levels.

Young people who are excluded and who go missing

Detached youth and community work has a long and established history of networking with young people on their streets, around their clubs and with their peer groups. The idea is to reach out to young people who are not attending centre-based activities either because they had been excluded or because they themselves felt that they did not 'fit in' (see Crimmens et al 2004 for further details of this).

Linking closely with the work of youth justice staff, social work and youth and community workers, the detached outreach work complements other provisions, engaging with the 'hard to reach'. As reviewed by Crimmens et al 2004 detached youth work plays an important role in engaging with those young people deemed to be 'anti social', 'beyond control' and 'difficult to engage'. Indeed, outreach detached youth work is an integral part of many crime prevention programmes (Crimmens et al 2004). The recent publication of the 'engaging youth enquiry' under the Nuffield Review of 14 to 19 education and training (Rathbone 2008) noted the importance of detached outreach youth work. It clarified that many of those young people who have histories of being looked after or of being in local authority often:

> have to be actively sought out by detached youth workers on street corners. ...
> These 'significant others' helped them to rejoin an increasingly complex

and confusing society. The detached youth workers we have worked with are extraordinary people: spend an evening with them on the streets of Manchester, Tower Hamlets or Hackney and you will quickly realise how skilled they are. They are successful because they have worked, often for years, in the same community building trust and local knowledge. Youth work really matters

(Rathbone 2008: 3–4)

The Ten Year Youth Strategy (DCSF 2007) and the government's 'respect action plan' (HO 2006c) focus on the five outcomes of Every Child Matters. In effort to secure the outcomes requested in the government's 'respect action plan' (HO 2006c), discussion of the role of detached outreach work needs to be placed firmly onto the agenda.

The essential principles of outreach are that they complement the work of centre-based activities, moving staff out from their familiar territory to spaces occupied by the young people themselves. This passes a message to the young people. It tells them that even if they are excluded from the centre base, their behaviour will be addressed. Essentially it is saying that the young person cannot be more powerful than the service that is there to support them.

This is important as it is their own uncontrolled and abandoned sense of power that is frightening for the young person to manage. This is not being patronising, but is recognising the severity of the problems that many of the young people are trying to cope with. The message of a continued outreach service is that 'anti-social behaviour' or, more importantly, the impact of multiple problems, is not beyond the remit of the adult professional community. This is an essential message to convey, one that is central to therapeutic outreach. The message is that the practitioners want to form an attachment with the young person, they want to engage with the young person's problems and help them to manage the impact of the problems. They have resources, often themselves as the strongest resource, that can help the young person to manage their behaviour.

This recognises that if a young person disrupts a centre-based resource, or runs away from support, they are demonstrating their own distress. The circumstances that they have to manage are, they feel, beyond their own and others' understanding and control.

Indeed, as noted by Kim, aged 16 who had a history of disruptive behaviour at school and youth service provision, running away meant a number of things. She frequently ran away from home and was in a particularly abusive relationship with her 'boyfriend' who was encouraging her to have sex with his friends in return for cigarettes and alcohol. For her, running away meant:

• Giving herself some space.
• Avoiding the stupid questions adults kept asking her.
• Forgetting the problems – leaving them behind.
• Just doing something – being in control.

(Kim, aged 16, Pearce et al 2009 forthcoming)

This suggests that the reasons for running away were complicated. They were both about:

- Trying to take some control.
- Giving herself some 'space' away from problems and questions about these problems.
- Trying to exert some control over her situation: exert some sense of agency rather than being a victim of events.

These sorts of complexities can be overlooked amongst the anxiety of dealing with a 'missing' case. The desire to find and return the young person – unfortunately often returning them to the situation that they ran away from – can dominate and the full assessment of the young person's therapeutic needs can be missed.

In fact, the missing component to work with missing young people is the question of why they ran away in the first place and what their therapeutic needs might be on return! The planned return to a place of safety may not include the provision of staff time and resources to reach out to the young person while they are missing or to assess the complex reasons of why they went missing. Therapeutic outreach advocates that this work takes place on an ongoing basis with vulnerable young people.

Pearce et al (2002) produced 10 key recommendations, the sixth arguing that 'therapeutic outreach' is used as an underlying approach to work with sexually exploited children and young people (Pearce et al 2002: 71). The term 'therapeutic outreach' was proposed by Margaret Rosemary, a supervisor who oversaw some of the supervision received by researchers.

Therapeutic outreach

This term breaks from the traditional understanding of therapeutic work where a 'patient' attends a regular appointment at a space 'owned' by a therapist. Many sexually exploited children and young people find it hard, if not impossible, to make or keep appointments. Others may feel uneasy or unable to remain within a closed room for a period of time. If the practitioners can see the young person on the street, at the café, the club, or drop-in centre – at places that are familiar and comfortable to the young person – a relationship might begin to develop. Indeed, many young people need the reassurance that the practitioner is going to put every effort into engaging with them, not only at times set by the practitioner, but at times when they felt the most need themselves.

Many of the young people's response to their experience of abusive or neglectful, inconsistent and unreliable adult carers is to push other adult carers away. To reject the offer of support before it is even made or explained! That is, the defence to previous abuse is to avoid attachment to any other adult for fear of further abuse, disappointment and pain.

Those young people who have entrenched problem drug and alcohol use are even harder to engage with as they are living more confused and chaotic lives than their drug-free counterparts. Problems such as going missing, running away, switching attachments from one peer group to another or/and from one adult to another are common for sexually exploited young people (Scott and Skidmore 2006). They are exaggerated by problem drug and alcohol use.

I return to this below when discussing ideas about attachment and engagement with the young people. For the moment, it is important to recognise that offering an appointment at a regular time each week in a place chosen by the practitioner may not be a successful method of engaging many sexually exploited children and young people. This does not mean that it is not achievable in the longer term, but that it is unlikely to be a model for initial engagement with the most damaged and disturbed young people. Therapeutic outreach is an intervention that aims to fill the gap between disrupted and planned engagement with sexually exploited children and young people.

Therapeutic outreach: Lessons from therapeutic communities

Childhood First (formerly the Peper Harow Foundation), a provider of therapeutic residential care for young people who had experienced difficulties or been damaged through past experiences of care (see www.childhoodfirst.org.uk for more details), specifically addresses how psychodynamic theories can inform work with young people who had experienced disrupted care plans.

The therapeutic community model recognised the importance of the integration of therapeutic thinking to the day-to-day experiences of the young person. The environment within which they live (the institution: be it family, foster or residential care), the adult carers they are in touch with (parents, foster carers of key workers) and the feelings of the young person at the time (their emotional state), are all equally important considerations to bear in mind when developing therapeutic support for the young person.

As such, the concept of therapy is extended from one that employs a one-hour meeting between patient and therapist in a quiet room, to one that embraces all aspects of day-to-day, night-by-night living. The 'noise' of everyday living becomes the reason and means for therapeutic intervention. When talking about the role of therapy within therapeutic communities, Ward notes that:

> ...the therapeutic work with young people is not confined just to the 'therapeutic hour' of planned individual sessions, nor to the equivalent in group work, family or community meetings, or in the classroom work. The therapeutic work is also potentially ongoing in all the other times and contexts in which the young person is involved, and especially in the course of everyday life and the social and other interactions which this entails
>
> (Ward 2003: 119)

What is important to note in Ward's comments above is that the one-to-one meetings and the group and family meetings continue, but they are a part of a broader therapeutic model of support. They are complemented by an approach that is responsive. They recognise the need to work with incidents as and when and where they arise, and to be vigilant, aware of the significance carried in each moment of contact with the young person.

Opportunity-led work

Ward continues to explain this as 'opportunity-led work': staff having the capacity to spot and use the opportunities that arise in everyday activities and exchanges between themselves and the young people they work with:

> There may be incidents or moments in everyday interactions ... it is in these moments, and with the sometimes fleeting feelings which they may engender, that some of the most useful work can be done. This is the work that I have called Opportunity Led work
>
> (Ward 2003: 121)

He distinguishes between reacting and responding to these events.

> [Reacting is] a hasty and un-thought-out way of dealing with situations, whereas by 'responding' I mean dealing with situations on the basis of a well thought through judgement
>
> (Ward 2003: 121)

Opportunity-led work involves four stages:

- Observation and assessment.
- Decision-making.
- Taking action.
- Closure.

The worker needs to be able to observe the behaviour of the young person and feel confident to make an (almost spontaneous) assessment of its meaning. They then need to be able to decide what to do and what actions these decisions involve. They then need to be able to close the intervention.

Closure might mean simply acknowledging that something has happened, something has been said and that it has not been possible to give a considered response there and then. This would mean that the worker and young person try to agree a way to follow up on the incident, either in the next hour, day, week, or over a longer time. Alternatively closure might mean that the young person and the worker feel that the incident has been resolved and that associated feelings are comfortable enough to be left.

Holding the young person in mind

This work links well with concepts advocated by Trieschman et al (1969) in their classic text about the 'other' 23 hours of life outside the one-hour therapy session. Although these authors assume that one hour of therapy is taking place, they also focus on what happens during the other 23 hours of life outside the counselor's room.

This work, along with the lessons that we can learn from opportunity-led therapeutic interventions described above, encourages awareness of the importance of holding the child in mind through sustained contact outside allocated appointment time. This is particularly important for work with young people who fail to make appointments or who go missing.

The spirit of therapeutic outreach – of holding the young person in mind wherever they are and of intending to go out to them, to reach out to them even if they do not respond – demonstrates conviction. The conviction is that the case will not be closed, that the behaviour can be managed and that it, or the young person, is not too powerful for the profession to address. This conviction can be reassuring to the young person. The feeling of having given up on themselves, or on others' ability to help them can be frightening. They might feel support from an approach that continues to try to contact them. When they return from running from home, it will be significant to them to know that practitioners were 'out there' looking for them, that they were held in someone's thinking while they were away.

Where is has been established, therapeutic outreach is advocated as an important component to the work with sexually exploited young people. As described in the Sheffield Sexual Exploitation Annual Report (2007) therapeutic outreach

> is the continual reaching out for a young person even though they may respond with silence and appear not to engage. This reaching out can be therapeutic in itself
>
> (Sheffield 2008)

When describing the need for flexible support, the project note that young people need the opportunity for:

> 'sounding off' (a need to be able to rant and complain), for 'popping in' (just need to know you're there when I need you) for 'outreach' (letters, texts, phone calls, active searching, visits) for 'crisis' (I need you to help me NOW), for 'holding' (staying with me where I am now) and for 'long term' (expecting nothing from them but constantly encouraging them)
>
> (Sheffield 2007: 10–11)

They continue:

> The young women often believe that they are better off looking after themselves due to poor experiences of parental or adult support and therefore need to see that their support worker is genuine and will walk

that extra mile for them before they are willing to engage. This can be incredibly demanding and emotionally draining which is why all workers have access to independent supervision

(Sheffield 2007: 10)

If the young person does not receive this message, and is left feeling that their emotions and circumstances are too dangerous and overpowering for anyone to manage, they are then left isolated, holding the anger and the burden of the abuse to themselves. The only answer is to run away, so that this escape becomes, by default, a reoccurring pattern and they will continue to run each time a crisis hits them.

As was noted in the Barnardos evaluation of service provision (Scott and Skidmore 2006) and in numerous other publications of work with sexually exploited young people (Melrose and Barrett 2004, Scott and Harper 2006) these young people's emotions, behaviours and circumstances are indeed difficult. However, the young people can be accessed, identified and worked with.

The Barnardos four 'A's

For this to happen, a good attachment to a supportive, non-abusive adult is central to recovery (Scott and Skidmore 2006: 48). According to Barnardos' work, this means working with the four 'A's:

- Access: 'considerable efforts are made to ensure that services are provided in a safe, attractive environment, flexible and responsive to young people's needs, by staff who take time to build a trusting relationship. Providing support to young people on their own terms is crucial, as is honesty about the boundaries of confidentiality'.
- Attention: ' ... attention that will "hook" a young person out of unsafe relationships into safe and positive ones. This entails focusing on the issues that mater to the young person and persistence over time'.
- Assertive outreach: 'establishing and maintaining contact is achieved through a range of methods, including regular texting, calls and cards, arranging to meet on the young person's "home ground" or at venues where they felt comfortable. The steady persistence of workers is eventually understood as being a genuine demonstration of concern and an indication of reliability. Such persistent engagement techniques are particularly important to counteract the influence of, often equally persistent, abusive adults'.
- Advocacy: ' ... our interviews with services and analysis of case histories have highlighted a number of factors which can act as "turning points" in young people's lives, where advocacy for the right kind of support at the right time can be particularly important ... '.

(Scott and Skidmore 2006: 48–49)

With such an extensive analysis of the needs of young people, and with a remit from government to engage with the most socially excluded young people, why is it that there is so little assertive, therapeutic outreach?

Is it purely a matter of resources: that there are inadequate funds for this work, or is it something to do with the challenges such work presents? While the lack of resources is a significant contributor, I want here to concentrate in more detail on the latter question. Is there something else about the work that pushes us away, that makes it really hard to achieve the perseverance necessary?

To follow up on this question, it is helpful to look at therapeutic ideas around attachment and relationship-based thinking to see how an understanding of this can inform work with sexually exploited children and young people.

Access and attachment: Relationship-based thinking

Making and maintaining contact with angry, depressed and disillusioned children can be hard. Doing the same with adolescents can be even more difficult, as they are asserting their right to experiment with their identity and their sexuality. They are living through the emotional and physical turmoil commonly associated with making the transition from child to adult (Coleman and Hendry 1999).

Many practitioners do not want to work with adolescents at all, let alone be faced with the complex issues brought to the fore by sexually exploited young people. Annie Hudson noted many social workers' reticence to work with young people, identifying a fear of the turmoil, anger and resistance that is evident in so many young people's lives (Hudson 1988). As noted in previous chapters, sexually exploited young men and women bring a range of different problems to be addressed. Pearce's study of 2002 noted that from a sample of 55 young women, 53 were regularly going missing, 39 had violent 'boyfriends', 34 were regularly self-harming, 30 had ongoing problems with heroin misuse, 22 had been raped, 18 had attempted suicide at least once, while only 3 had diagnosed mental health problems (Pearce et al 2002: 63). These were young women who were difficult to engage, difficult to maintain regular contact with and hard to provide for. Practitioners described them as:

> Lying, uncooperative, difficult to engage, unreliable, aggressive and abusive
> (Pearce et al 2002: 63)

Similarly, the two-year evaluation of Barnardo's services noted the difficult problems presented by the 42 (35 young women and 7 young men) in-depth case studies analysed:

> self harm or attempted suicide was identified in ten cases. The most recurrent issue discussed was the poor self regard in which young people held themselves ... a striking feature was the prevalence of various forms of

violence and abuse within the young people's families. The majority were form extremely disadvantaged backgrounds and had suffered sexual abuse in childhood (identified in 28 cases). ... In addition, domestic violence was known to have featured in 13 parental relationships, parental mental health problems were identified in 5 case studies, significant bereavement in 4, and parental alcohol/drug misuse in 14 cases

(Scott and Skidmore 2006: 29)

The point here is that trying to develop and maintain an attachment with these young people can feel challenging, if not impossible. Challenging behaviour is a sign of distress and should be a reason for continuing to try to engage, rather than the reason to let go. The generic, universal services designed for adolescents may assume behviours ascribed to a chronological age assessment. However, many vulnerable, damaged or abused young people may not have had the scope to develop age-appropriate maturity. It is argued that practitioners need to take a developmental perspective that looks not at the young person's chronological age, but at their developmental age: the stage that they have reached in their psychological development (Macfie et al 2001: 250).

The essence here is that if the young person has experienced disrupted or damaging early attachments to a parent or care giver, they may have little experience of how to manage stress and anxiety. The intervention from the practitioner may be about trying to 'rework' the young person's understanding of a relationship. All too often the harsh reality for workers experiencing constant rejection, aggression and abuse is that the impact of such rejection has to be hidden from view. There are too few forums for staff to 'tell it like it is' – to explore how working with the young people makes them feel and how they manage these feelings.

Attachments and the role of good attachments

Good enough early attachments between child and parent/carer help the child to see that anxiety and stress can be managed. Indeed, the basic premise is that the adult carer absorbs the anxious or distressed feelings expressed by the child, holds them and translates them into feelings that can then be understood and managed. If the child has not had this support through earlier years of development, and has also experienced adult carers being unable to manage their own feelings themselves, the child's development of an integrated self may be held back. Their developmental age will not match their chronological age and support and treatment will need to adapt to meet the child's developmental stage (for more information on attachment theory and its use in work with adolescents see Fonagy 2002).

Within a developmental perspective, young people's psychological make-up is seen to be developed within the context of close relationships. Working with this premise, relationship-based interventions are appropriate. Referring to 'the other' as the young person, Howe notes that:

... Practitioners must therefore be highly attuned and responsive ... they have to amplify what they feel and perceive in the other, in the manner of a secure parent – child relationship, to ensure as much emotional and psychological information is conveyed to the other who is not used to receiving so much interest and feedback in the context of a safe relationship

(Howe 2005: 218)

Disassociation

In work on child abuse and neglect, the 'blocking out' of feeling is a coping mechanism for a child who has been neglected and/or abused (Fonagy 2002). Fonagy refers to this 'disassociation', as a means through which children and young people develop psychological processes that help them to separate from pain, to avoid the associated thinking and feeling. Young people's self-harming behaviours, for example, or extensive drug or alcohol abuse (behaviours common to sexually exploited children and young people) can be a useful distraction, or disassociation from pain. In itself it can be a means of anaesthetising pain. If, as a child, banging your head against a wall helped to reduce the impact of other pains, cutting yourself as an adolescent might follow as a coping mechanism.

Similarly, if withdrawing, or running away from feeling and contact with abusers was a mechanism for coping in the past, the adolescent will continue to run from home when stressed or frightened.

Developing a good attachment: Avoidance and defence

If a child or young person is beginning to make a good attachment to a practitioner or carer, this may be taking them into unfamiliar and frightening territory. They might feel overwhelmed at the very moment of beginning engagement; at the very moment that a worker felt they were 'getting somewhere'. The developing feelings might be too unfamiliar, frightening and overpowering for the young person to manage. The young person may be fearful that a good thing will be short lived, that patterns of the past will be repeated and that anything good will be short lived and that they will be abandoned and disappointed.

Also, if a good relationship does actually work, it means that they will have to stop, settle, account for themselves, and, at a deeper level, trust someone else with the feelings that they have split of and run away from for many years. Indeed, the young person might be defended from starting a good relationship as this could mean they have to face the fact that they are unhappy and depressed.

Fonagy considers the meaning and applicability of concepts such as denial and avoidance in his work on therapeutic work with adolescents (Fonagy 2002). There is a plethora of work that explores psychodynamic work with young people (Pooley and Worthington 2003). For now, it is helpful to refer to the fear that can be created for a young person in the process of forming a good attachment to a practitioner. Howe notes that attachment-based support:

> In the case of insecure children, the availability and sensitivity of carers at times of need is not so straightforward … Displays of weakness, dependency, need and vulnerability in the self or others makes them anxious, avoidant and rejecting.
>
> (Howe 2005: 215–16)

Often, because of previous negative experiences of contact with statutory services including education, housing, child protection services and police, these young people may have little confidence in the stability of relationships that support services are offering. Staff burnout, high case loads and the threat of withdrawal of funding often means that staff feel that it might be irresponsible to commit to longer-term interventions.

I argue that there is not enough consideration put into the important contribution that a relationship can make to the sexually exploited young person. The Nuffield 'Engaging Youth Enquiry' (Rathbone 2008) noted that young people:

> talked at length of the importance of working with a 'significant adult', often a youth worker or a connexions adviser. This does not mean an occasional conversation but a sustained relationship. These professionals do not take the place of parents … but they provide a point of contact, someone who will listen to them ' … they are absolutely crucial for these young people who find themselves without parents and in care homes … '
>
> (Rathbone 2008: 3–4)

The work with sexually exploited young people can illustrate how hard it is for some young people to even contemplate being available for a relationship, let alone develop one.

For example, Sue, aged 18 years, believed it was too late for her to use any support. She had had a series of different key workers and social workers whilst in care. She fluctuated between feeling that she was being passed around between workers and running away from them. Similarly, Iona, aged 17 years, explained that she had a meeting with the AA that evening but that she felt too low to manage the journey: 'I'm too depressed and the journey takes too long' (Pearce et al 2002: 64).

Nine of 20 young women who had serious problems with heroin use were trying to cut down on their use, trying to attend drop-in sessions with local drugs workers, but were anxious about the implications of keeping an appointment. For example, Jo, aged 16 years, finally agreed to make an appointment to see the community drugs team and the doctor. On the day of the appointment she came to the sexual exploitation project saying that she had stayed out all night at her friend's flat and that she had 'drunk her head off'. She had a severe headache and did not want to talk to drugs workers. Later, she recognised that she got so drunk because she was anxious about the appointment. She wanted help, but was afraid that getting help meant having to face up to her problems. She knew that the drugs worker wanted to form a relationship with her, but she was afraid that the relationship would mean that someone would ask her to commit to working with them and trust them (Pearce et al 2007: 64).

Silence and time: Letting feelings and awareness come in their own time

This brings me now to look at some of the implications for the young person of making and sustaining a relationship. As I have argued, my point is that it is through being part of a supportive relationship that the young person can both address their depression, and also experience a model of how attachment can be helpful, rather than damaging. This experience of a model of 'good' relationship suggests how other good relationships might be developed in the future.

As noted by many practitioners however, this process is not straightforward. If the young person is running away, they might be finding it difficult, if not impossible, to talk. Long periods may pass when the young person just wants to test the relationship, project their feelings on the worker so that the worker feels as depressed, as chaotic and confused as they do. They may challenge the suggestion that anything can ever improve, or that they will ever be in any different place or situation than that of the present.

In a fascinating and extremely helpful analysis of counselling work in schools titled 'Feeling like crap: young people and the meaning of self esteem', Luxmoore (2008: 115) draws on his work as a therapeutic counsellor in schools with disaffected young people, to note that:

> faced with the future, many young people regress. When the past has been chaotic, full of insecure attachments, broken promises and lies, they have to go back before they can go forward ... By the time they're sixteen, they've all been shocked by the death of someone they knew. They've been reminded of their own potential to die. So, describing the future as a safe, linear progression (if you do that, this will happen and if you do this, that will happen) may convince some but for most it makes no sense because it avoids the really big questions: Will I matter? Will I be loved? Will there be any point in my life?

He refers to a conversation assessed in supervision, between a counsellor and a 16-year-old young man. The young man did not know what he wanted to do in the future or what could help him to find a path forward. The counsellor realised in supervision that:

> ... If he could speak he'd probably say that it's important to be liked –
> liked by his family, liked by his friends and even, possibly, loved by them.
> Then the immediate future would still be unclear but, in the long run, he'd
> be all right.

And that as a counsellor:

> ... she realises that he's telling the truth. He really doesn't know. She tries
> to think what to say that will be helpful but feels at a loss. 'I feel bad' she
> says, 'just leaving it like that'
>
> (Luxmoore 2008: 155)

I choose this extract for two reasons.

Firstly, it is often the case that the young person does not know how to talk
about what is important to them. In this case referred to by Luxmoore, the
counsellor does not force the question, but allows the silence to remain. There
has been much discussion of the use of silences in psychodynamic work (see
Fonagy 2002 for more detail) but in general, silences can feel uncomfortable. It
can feel as though they should be filled, rather than allow them to speak their
own meanings.

The need for a 'quick' improvement in behaviour, the idea that a young
person can be referred to a project and that improvements in behaviour can be
visible after one or two months' intervention dramatically underestimates the
impact of abuse and exploitation on the young person. That is, the young
people need time and support to identify what they cannot say as much as what
they can say. They need to be able to hear their own silences within a developing secure relationship and to realise what they can or cannot talk about. All
of this takes time, and only happens as an attachment is being made between
the worker and the young person.

Secondly, the extract touches on the impotence of the worker to help. 'I feel
bad, just leaving it like that'. This goes straight to the frustration felt by many
project workers when faced with the reality that they cannot 'rescue' or
'change' young people, 'create' different lives for them.

A final example from practice looks at the need for the worker to allow time
and space for the young person to begin to address the feelings that are difficult
for them. I refer to an incident that took place between myself and Mark, a
sexually exploited young man aged 15 years. I was working on a sexual health
awareness programme in a youth justice project, and had a number of one-to-
one meetings with Mark, who had been referred to the Youth Offending Team
project for stealing from a neighbour. The details of his offence were well
known within the locality and were dismissed as insignificant. They were seen
to have little long-term importance as they resulted from petty neighbourly
rivalry and were demonstrative of deeper problems Mark was experiencing.
The more important worry was that Mark was developing a sexual relationship
with an older man who was known locally for having a problem with heroin

use, for dealing in a variety of drugs and for having inappropriate sexual relationships with young men.

Mark and I were sitting next to each other in the project building. We were reading a magazine about health issues for young people. We were getting on well, talking about the various entries to the magazine and relating them to the lives of young people. There was an entry about plastic surgery and breast enlargements and the associated health hazards. Mark asked me, with a genuine honesty, why it was that any man should be attracted to women at all. This was not a flippant question. There was no embarrassment or 'wind up' going on. It had felt like a safe moment for him to express his confusion about why boys should be attracted to girls.

Of course he was asking for much more. He wanted the opportunity to open up a conversation about sex, sexuality and sexual orientation. This might have led to us discussing some aspect of his potential or actual relationship with the older man.

A silence developed while he was, I think, considering what he had said and how he felt about it. I felt uncomfortable with the silence and felt the need to speak. I claimed that boys should not have to like girls as a matter of course. People should be free to develop intimate relationships with the same sex, to be sexually attracted to the same sex.

Rather than respond to what I had said, Mark looked as though his train of thought had been broken. He changed the subject to the topic of the next page of the magazine and the subject was closed between us.

Referring back to 'opportunity-led intervention', an opportunity had arisen, and rather than giving time for it to be understood, I reacted to my own needs to be seen to be supportive. I had closed down Mark's train of thought and prevented him from speaking further. There had not been a decision made about how to follow up on the opportunity, to assess what action to take, or how to close the topic so that we both felt it had been contained.

This project had an established supervision structure that encouraged each worker to discuss difficult issues both within group and individual supervision. The team focused on the exchange between Mark and myself. We role-played different responses that I could have made, looking at how the conversation could have developed if I had responded differently. I was supported in individual supervision to explore my own attitudes to adolescence, sexuality and sexual orientation. I realised that I had reacted to a fear that I might not manage what Mark was trying to tell me or that I might not be able to support him in exploring his sexuality.

I was supported to understand that moments such as this one between Mark and myself do pass, some being managed well and others not so well. I was able to return to work with Mark feeling that I had learnt from the experience. This was unusual. Invariably workers are left with feelings of disappointment and confusion, anger or regret. These feelings then impact on the way that the relationship with the young person continues. The longer-term implications are that the workers either become rejecting, being fearful of returning to the young person, or may become 'stuck' in an inappropriate role with the young person, perhaps in the role of mother, father, friend or enemy, repeating dangerous patterns of the past without an analysis that breaks repeating cycles (see transference and counter-transference below).

Supervision: Caring for the worker

The need for good and regular supervision of practitioners' work is identified in the example above. All too often one isolated worker is receiving referrals and being expected to engage, manage and respond to young people's very challenging behaviour without any supervision, either at a personal or professional level. This is a recipe for burn-out. Remarkably, a number of projects have survived through the dedication of one or two 'pioneers' (Jago and Pearce 2008) but this can be at the expense of the welfare of the worker and then, in consequence, the welfare of the child.

For the worker to carry the burden of accessing, engaging, listening and intervening with the traumas presented by the young people in a way that is meaningful and focused on sustaining longer-term change, they must be supported themselves.

If displacement, or projection of feelings from the young person to the practitioner continue uninterrupted, familiar patterns will continue to repeat themselves. This will be to the detriment of both the practitioner and the young person. Wilson highlights the importance of good supervision to maintaining appropriate and supportive interventions with young people, particularly those who carry multiple problems and challenging behaviour (Wilson 2003). He refers to supervision as a safeguard, a framework that helps staff to achieve their aims.

Above all, supervision safeguards this structure, taking care that staff are doing and are helped to be doing what they are supposed to be doing (Wilson 2003: 220). If the practitioner is not supported, they can be overwhelmed with both the young person's feelings and their own feelings experienced in response. Indeed, this may well be happening for workers who had not intended to engage with therapeutic work or who had not received any training in helping them to understand the implications of asking particular questions or exploring certain behaviours in depth. This can mean that rather than addressing potentially painful subjects, staff may avoid asking the questions that need to be asked, or may ask and then feel overwhelmed and unable to help the young person.

Finally, I want to look at one of the issues that can emerge in good supervision for practitioners working with sexually exploited children and young people in more detail.

Transference and counter-transference

It has been established that therapeutic work with clients involves the therapist understanding and working with the projections, the transferences and counter-transferences that take place as a central part of the therapeutic relationship (Bateman et al 2002). Greenson describes transference as:

> The experience of feelings, drives, attitudes, fantasies and defences towards a person in the present, which do not befit that person but are a repetition of reactions originating in regard to significant persons of early childhood, unconsciously displaced onto figures in the present. The two outstanding characteristics of a transference reaction are: it is repetition and it is inappropriate
>
> (Greenson 1967: 155 in Bateman et al 2002: 52)

Much more work could be done to explore the way that young people project their feelings about significant adults, such as their mother or father, onto the sexual exploitation worker with whom they develop a relationship. If the workers find themselves being idolised as the good mother or father that the young person has been yearning for, or hated as an evil enemy, they need help and support in keeping this in perspective. Good supervision is needed to help the practitioner express and understand what is happening so that the young person's ideals are not shattered and unrealistic expectations are not upheld.

For further information about the meaning and application of these concepts to work with young people, see Pooley and Worthington 2003. For here, it is important to note that such transferences can be damaging if they remain at the unconscious level and if practitioners are not supported to identify and work with them.

Conclusion

In this chapter I have identified some of the contributions that therapeutic thinking can make to the work with sexually exploited children and young people.

Such approaches help us to think about why a young person might run away, what running actually means for them. It helps us to understand why it takes a young person a long time to establish a relationship with a worker, and why that relationship may, on occasions, break down. When practitioners feel attacked, confused and chaotic in their attempts to engage with and listen to the young people, therapeutic support might help them to see that these are feelings projected by the young person. The worker is, in effect, feeling the feelings that the young person holds. When the worker feels helpless, angry, abandoned and frustrated, these are also emotions experienced by the young person. How this is managed and worked with in the developing relationship with the young person is important. An understanding of some of the therapeutic concepts developed in psychodynamic interventions can help develop this understanding and underpin the need for good supervision of staff engaged in this work.

Projects providing dedicated and specialist interventions with sexually exploited young people need support so that workers are not left feeling isolated, left alone to carry a 'pile of pain' (as one young person put it). Providing support for the worker offers a model for the worker to use when giving support to the young people.

Failing to address these needs passes a message that the young people and the problems they carry are either too hard to be managed or not significant enough to call for sustained support. These messages, whether conveyed consciously or unconsciously, are damaging and must be challenged. Supported practice that understands the importance of good relationships in the young person's lives will be able to match the development of instrumental/concrete resources (such as educational services, youth work trips out and activities, child protection structures and procedures) with a delivery that touches the internal worlds of the young people concerned.

Bibliography

Aapola, S., Gonick, M., Harris, A. (2005) *Young Femininity: Girlhood, Power and Social Change*. Palgrave: Basingstoke.

ACPO (1997a) *Guidelines in Relation to Coercers, Users and Victims of Prostitution of Children*. London: ACPO.

—— (1997b) *Guidelines in Relation to Coercers, Users and Victims of Prostitution of Children*. London: ACPO.

—— (2004) *Policing Prostitution : ACPOs Policy, Strategy and Operational Guidelines for Dealing with Exploitation and Abuse through Prostitution*. London: ACPO.

—— (2005a) *Guidance on the Management Recording and Investigation of Missing Persons*. Hampshire: The National Centre for policing excellence on behalf of the Association of Chief Police Officers.

—— (2005b) *Investigating Child Abuse and Safeguarding Children*. London: ACPO.

—— (2005c) *Guidance on the Management, Recording and Investigation of Missing Persons*. London: ACPO.

Adam, B., Beck, U., Van Loon, J. (2000) *The Risk Society and Beyond: Critical Issues for Social Theory*. London: Sage.

Aggleston, P., Hurry, J., Warwick, I. (2000) *Young People and Mental Health*. Wiley: Chichester.

Aitchinson, P., O'Brien, R. (1997) 'Redressing the balance: the legal context of child prostitution', in Barrett, D. (ed.) *Child Prostitution in Britain*. pp. 32–59. London: The Children's Society.

Alder, C., Worrall, A. (2004) *Girls' Violence: Myths and Realities*. New York: SUNNY Press.

Aldgate, J. Tunstill, J. (1994) *Implementing Section 17 of the Children Act- the First 18 Months*. Leicester, Leicester University, School of Social Work in Lee, M., O'Brien, R. (1995) *The Game's Up: Redefining Child Prostitution*. London: The Children's Society.

Allan, J. (2004) 'Mother blaming: a covert practice in therapeutic intervention'. *Australian Journal of Social Work*, 57(1):57–70.

Amos, V., Parmar, P. (1981) 'Resistance and responses: the experiences of black girls in Britain', in McRobbie, A., McCabe, T. (eds), *Feminism for Girls: An Adventure Story*. London: Routledge and Keegan Paul.

Anderson, B., O'Connell-Davidson, J. (2003) *Is Trafficking a Demand Led Problem?* Geneva: IOM.

Anon (2000) *Street Matters Project*. Available from: www.nspcc.org.uk (accessed 27 April 2009).

Awaken Project (2007a) *Annual Report.* Awaken Project, Blackpool Central Police Office, Bonny Street, Blackpool.

—— (2007b) *Conference presentation.* Available from: www.popcentre.org/conference/conferencepapers/2007/sexual_exploitation.pdf (accessed 20 April 2009).

Ayre, P., Barrett, D. (2000) 'Young people and prostitution: an end to the beginning'. *Children and Society,* 14:48–59.

Bailey, R., Blake, M. (1975) *Radical Social Work.* London: Edward Arnold.

Barkham, P. (2005) 'Journey through Britain's Muslim divide'. *The Guardian,* 16 July, 6–7.

Barn, R. (1993) *Black Children in the Care System.* London: Batsford/BAAF.

Barn, R., Andrew, L., Mantovani, V. (2005) *Life after Care. A Study of the Experiences of Young People from Different Ethnic Minority Groups.* York: JRF The Policy Press.

Barnard, M., McKeganey, N. (1996) *Sex Work on the Streets.* Milton Keynes: Open University Press.

Barnard, M., McKeganey, N., Bloor, M. (1990) 'A risky business'. *Community Care,* 5 July, 26–7.

Barnardos (1998) *Whose Daughter Next? Children Abused Through Prostitution.* London: Barnardo's.

—— (2002) *Stolen Childhood: Barnardos Work with Children Abused Through Prostitution.* Barkingside: Barnardos.

—— (2008) www.barnardos.org.uk/ethical.pdf (accessed 21 April 2009).

—— (2009) *Barnardos Statement of Ethical Research Practice.* Available from: www.barnarods.org.uk/resources (accessed 21 April 2009).

Barnardo's (2000) *Things We Don't Talk About.* London: Barnardos.

Barnardos Young Men's Project (2004) 'Workshop on working with young men'. *Young People and Sexual Exploitation Conference.* Brighton: The Trust for the Study of Adolescence.

Barrett, D. (ed.) (1997) *Child Prostitution in Britain: Dilemmas and Practical Responses.* London: The Children's Society.

Barter, C. (1996) *Nowhere to Hide: Giving Young Runaways a Voice.* London: Centrepoint.

Barter, C. et al (2004) *Peer Violence in Children's Residential Care.* Palgrave: Macmillan.

Bateman, A., Brown, D., Pedder, J. (2000) *Introduction to Psychotherapy: An Outline of Psychodynamic Principles and Practice.* London: Routledge.

—— (2002) *Introduction to Psychotherapy: An Outline of Psychodynamic Principles and Practice.* Sussex: Brunner Routledge.

Beck, U. (1992) *Risk Society: Towards a New Modernity.* London: Sage.

Beckett, C., Macey, M. (2001) 'Race, gender and sexuality: the oppression of multiculturalism'. *Women's Studies International Forum,* 24; 3(4):309–319.

Blake, S., Butcher, J. (2005) 'Young men and participation: Alcohol and other drugs and sexual risk taking . *WYM Working with Young Men,* 4(2):6–9.

Blake, S., Muttock, S. (2004) *Assessment, Evaluation and Sex and Relationships Education: A Practical Toolkit for Education, Health and Community Settings.* London: National Children's Bureau.

Boswell, G. (2000) *Violent Children and Adolescents Asking the Questions Why.* London: Whur.

Brain, T., Duffin, T., Anderson, S., Parchment, P. (1998) *Child Prostitution: A Report on the ACPO Guidelines and Pilot Studies in Wolverhampton and Nottinghamshire.* Gloucester: Gloucestershire Constabulary.

Breuil, B. (2008) 'Precious children in a heartless world. The complexities of child trafficking in Marseille'. *Children and Society*, 22(3):223–234.

British Society of Criminology (2005) *Code of Ethics for Researchers in the Field of Criminology*. Available from: www.britsoccrim.org/ethical.htm (accessed 14 March 2007).

Brooks, P. (1994) *Psychoanalysis and Story Telling*. Oxford: Blackwell.

Brooks-Gordon, B. (2006) *The Price of Sex: Prostitution, Policy and Society*. Devon: Willan Publishing.

Brown, A. (2004) *Children and Society*. 18:344–354. Available from: www.interscience. wiley.com (accessed 21 April 2009).

Brown, K. (2004) *Paying the Price: A Consultation Paper on Prostitution- Consultation Response from the National Youth Campaign on Sexual Exploitation*. London: The Children's Society.

—— (2006) 'Participation and young people involved in prostitution'. *Child Abuse Review*, 15(5):294–312.

Browne, K., Hamilton, C. (1998) 'Physical violence between young adults and their parents'. *Adolescents with a History of Child Maltreatment*, 13(1):59–79.

Bryon, T. (2008) *Safer Children in a Digital World. The Report of the Bryon Review*. Nottingham: Department of Children, Schools and Families Publications.

Brooks-Gordon, B. (2006) *The Price of Sex: Prostitution, Policy and Society*. Devon: Willan Publishing.

Campbell, R., O'Neill, M. (2006) *Sex Work Now*. Devon: Willan Publishing.

Carell, T. (2000) *Working with Parents of Aggressive Children a Practitioners Guide*. Washington: The American Psychological Association.

Centrepoint (1997) *Centre Point Annual Report 1996-1997: Getting Out of Boxes*. London: Centre point.

CEOP (2006) *Understanding Online Social Network Services and Risks to Youth: Stakeholders Perspectives*. London: CEOP.

—— (2008) *thinkuknow*. Available from: www.thinkuknow.co.uk (accessed 23 March 2009).

CEOP, HO, BIA (2007) *A Scoping Project on Child Trafficking in The UK*. London: CEOP, HO, BIA.

Chase, E., Statham, J. (2004) *The Commercial Sexual Exploitation of Children and Young People: An Overview of Key Literature and Data*. London: Thomas Coram Research Unit, Institute of Education, University of London.

—— (2005) 'Commercial and sexual exploitation of children and young people in the UK: A review'. *Child Abuse Review*, 14:4–25.

Children's and Young People's Participation Learning Network (2009) Available from: www.uwe.ac.uk/solar/ChildParticipationNetwork/Home.htm (accessed 23 March 2009).

Clarke, J., Critcher, C., Johnson, R. (1979) *Working Class Culture: Studies in History and Theory*. London: Hutchinson.

Coleman, J. (2007) 'Emotional health and wellbeing', in *Adolescence and Health*. pp. 41–61. Chichester: Wiley.

Coleman, J., Brooks, F. (2009) *Kay Data on Adolescence 2006–2008*. Brighton: Trust for the Study of Adolescence.

Coleman, L., Cater, S. (2005) *Underage 'Risky' Drinking: Motivations and Outcomes*. York: Joseph Rowntree Foundation and Brighton: Trust for the Study of Adolescence.

Coleman, J., Hagel, A. (2007) 'The nature of risk and resilience in adolescence', in —— (eds) (2008) *Adolescence, Risk and Resilience: Against the Odds*. pp. 1–17. Wiley series in understanding adolescence. Chichester: Wiley.

Coleman, J., Hendry, L. (1999) *The Nature of Adolescence*. London: Routledge.

Coleman, J., Scofield, J. (2005) *Key Data on Adolescence*. 5th Edition. Brighton: Trust for the Study of Adolescence.

—— (2007) *Key Data on Adolescence*. 6th Edition. Brighton: Trust for the Study of Adolescence.

Coffey, A. (1999) *The Ethnographic Self: Fieldwork and the Representation of Identity*. London: Sage Publications.

Community Care (2008) *DCSF Sets Out Remit For Child Protection Review*. Available from: www.communitycare.co.uk/Articles/2008/11/17/109999/baby-p-balls-calls-on-laming-to-examine-legal-barriers-to-care.html (accessed 21 April 2009).

Connor, D.F. (2002) *Agression and Anti-Social Behaviour in Children & Adolescents*. London: Guildford Press.

Cook, D., Burton, M., Robinson, A. (2004) *Evaluation of Specialist Domestic Violence Courts/Fast Track Systems*. London: CPS, DCA, CJS.

Cooper, A., Lousada, J. (2005) *Borderline Welfare: Feeling and Fear of Feeling in Modern Welfare*. London: Karnac Books.

Cornwall, A., Lindisfarne, N. (1994) *Dislocating Masculinity: Comparative Ethnographies*. London: Routledge.

Cottew, G., Oyefeso, A. (2005) 'Illicit drug use among Bangladeshi women living in the United Kingdom: An exploratory qualitative study of a hidden population in East London'. *Drugs: Education, Prevention and Policy*, 12(3):171–188.

Council of Europe (2005) *Convention on Action against Trafficking in Human Beings*. Warsaw: Council of Europe.

—— (2007) *Council of Europe Convention on the Protection of Children against Sexual Exploitation and Sexual Abuse*. Available from: www.coe.int (accessed 23 March 2009).

Coy, M. (2006) 'This morning I'm a researcher, this afternoon I'm an outreach worker ethical dilemmas in practitioner research'. *International Journal of Social Research Methodology*, 9(5):419–431.

—— (2007) 'Young women, local authority care and selling sex: findings from research'. *British Journal of Social Work*. Advanced access published August 20th 2007, Oxford University Press on behalf of the British Association of Social Workers.

Craig, G (2008) 'Special Issue'. *Child Slavery Worldwide*, 22(3):147–149.

Crimmens, D., Factor, F., Jeffs, T., Pitts, J., Pugh, C., Spence, J., Turner, P. (2004) *Reaching Socially Excluded Young People: A National Study of Street-based Youth Work*. Leicester: National Youth Agency.

Crosby, S., Barrett, D. (1999) 'Poverty and youth prostitution: A case study', in *Young People, Drugs and Community Safety*. pp. 127–134. Lyme Regis: Russell House Publishing.

Crown Prosecution Service/Department of Health/Home Office (2005) *Provision of Therapy for Child Witnesses Prior to a Criminal Trial: Practice Guidance*. London: CPS.

Crown Prosecution Service (2006) *Children and Young People: CPS Policy on Prosecuting Criminal Cases Involving Children and Young People as Victims and Witnesses*. London: CPS.

Croydon (2008) *Croydon Safeguarding Children Board (CSCB): Keeping Croydon Safe for Children Annual Report 2007-2008*. London: London Borough of Croydon.

Currie, C. (ed.) (2004) *Health Behaviour in School Aged Children (HBSC) Study: International Report for the 2001/2002 Survey*. Copenhagen: WHO.

Cusick, L. (2002) 'Youth prostitution: A literature review'. *Child Abuse Review*, 11:230–251.

Cusick, L., Martin, A., May, T. (2003) *Vulnerability and Involvement in Drug Use and Sex Work*. Home Office Research Study 268. London: Her Majesties Stationary Office.

Darch, T. (2004) 'Terence Higgins Trust West Street Team; working with young men', in Melrose, M. (ed.), with Barrett D. 2004. *Op Cit.* pp. 92–102.

Davies, P., Feldman, R. (1992) Selling sex in Cardiff and London, in Aggleton, P. (ed.) *Men Who Sell Sex; International Perspectives on Male Prostitution and AIDS*. London: UCL Press.

—— (1997) 'Prostitute men now', in Scambler, G., Scambler, A. (eds) *Rethinking Prostitution: Purchasing Sex in the 1990's*. London: Routledge.

Denzins, N. (1968) 'Communications: On the ethics of disguised observation'. *Social Problems*, 15:502–504.

Department of Children Schools and Families (2007) *Aiming High For Young People: A Ten Year Strategy For Positive Activities*. London: HM Treasury and DCSF.

—— (2008a) *Children and Young People in Mind*. The final report of the national CAMHs review. London: Department of Health.

—— (2008b) *Government Response to the Report by the Sex and Relationship Education (SRE) Review Steering Group*. London: HMG.

—— (2008c) *Reducing the Number of Young People not in Education, Employment or Training (NEET) by 2013*. DCSF 00294 3. Available from: www.dcsf.gov.uk/14-19/documents/NEET%20%20strategy.pdf (accessed 23 March 2009).

—— (2008d) *Safeguarding Children in a Digital World: Developing a LSCB e-Safety Strategy*. London: DCSF.

—— (2008e) *Safeguarding Children and Young People Who May Have Been Trafficked*. London: DCSF.

—— (2008f) *Delivering 14 to 19 Reform: Next Steps. A Commitment from the Children's Plan*. London: DCSF.

—— (2008g) *Staying Safe: Action Plan*. DCSF: London.

—— (2009) *Safeguarding Children and Young People from Sexual Exploitation*. London: DCSF.

Department of Communities and Local Government (2005) *Sustainable Communities: Settled Homes, Changing Lives*. London: DCLG, HMSO.

—— (2007a) *English House Condition Survey Headline Report 2006*. London: CLG.

—— (2007b) *Tackling Youth Homelessness: Briefing Paper 18*. HMG West Yorkshire. Available from: www.communities.gov.uk (accessed 23 March 2009).

—— (2008) *Statutory Homelessness Statistics*. London: CLG.

Department for Education and Skills (2004a) *Every Child Matters: Change for Children*. London: HMSO. Available from: www.dfes.gov.uk (accessed 23 March 2009).

—— (2004b) *Sex and Relationship Guidance* (update). Available from: www.dfes.gov.uk (accessed 23 March 2009).

—— (2004c) *Children Looked After by Local Authorities, Year Ending 31 March 2003, Volume 2: Local Authority Tables*. Available from: www.defs.gov.uk/DB/VOL?V000454/finalvolume1.pdf (accessed 23 March 2009).

—— (2005) *Youth Matters*. London: HMSO. Available from: www.dfes.gov.uk (accessed 23 March 2009).

Department of Health (2005a) *Victims of Violence and Abuse Prevention Programme: Prostitution, Pornography and Trafficking Group*. London: Department of Health.

—— (2005b) *New Operational Procedures for NHS RECs: Guidance for Applicants to Research Ethics Committees*. London: Department of Health.

Department of Health/Home Office (2000) *Safeguarding Children Involved in Prostitution: Supplementary Guidance to Working Together to Safeguard Children*. Department of Health, Home Office, Department of Education and Employment, National Assembly for Wales. London: HMSO.

—— (2001) *National Plan for Safeguarding Children from Commercial Exploitation*. Available from: www.dh.gov.uk (accessed 23 March 2009).

Department of Health/NIMHE (2008) 'Victims of violence and abuse prevention programme'. Published in association with NIMHE, HO, Ministry of Justice, DCSF, CEOP, NW Public Health Observatory, WHO, Royal Colleges, 3rd sector bodies.

Dickson, S. (2004) *Sex in the City: Mapping Commercial Sex across London*. London: The Poppy Project.

Dobash, R.E., Dobash, R.P. (2005) 'Abuser programmes and violence against women', in Smeenk, Malsch (eds) *Family Violence and Police Response: Learning From Research, Policy and Practice in European Countries*. England: Ashgate.

Dobash, R.E., Dobash, R.P., Cavanagh, K., Lewis, R. (2000) *Changing Violent Men*. Sage series on violence against women. London: Sage Publications.

Dodsworth, J. (2000) *Child Sexual Exploitation/Child Prostitution*. Social Work Monographs, 178. Norwich: University of East Anglia.

Donovan, K. (1991). *Hidden from View; An Explanation of the Little-Known World of Young Male Prostitutes in Great Britian and Europe*. London: Home Office and West Midland Police.

Dottridge, M. (2002) 'Trafficking in children in West and Central Africa'. *Gender and Development*, 10(1):38–49.

Dowling, S., Moreton, K., Wright, L. (2007) *Trafficking For the Purposes of Labour Exploitation: A Literature Review*. Home Office Report 10/07. London: Home Office.

Downey, L. (1997) 'Adolescent violence: A systemic and feminist perspective'. *Australian and New Zealand Journal of Family Therapy*, 18(2):70–79.

Drinkwater, S., Greenwood, H., with Melrose, M. (2004) 'Young people exploited through prostitution: A literature review', in Melrose, M. (ed.) with Barrett, D. 2004. *Op Cit.* pp. 23–35.

Driscoll, M., Ungoed-Thomas, J., Foggo, D. (2008) 'How many more baby Ps are there?' *The Sunday Times*, 16 November 2008.

ECPAT International (2008) *Consultative Meeting on Engaging Men and Boys in Combating Sexual Exploitation of Children and Adolescents*. Available from: www.ecpat.net/worldcongressIII/PDF/Publications/CSR/Thematic_Paper_CSR_ENG.pdf (accessed 21 April 2009).

ECPAT UK (2007) *'Missing out'. A study of child trafficking in the North West, North East and West Midlands*. London: ECPAT.

ESRC (2006) *Research Ethics Framework (REF)*. London: ESRC.

Eversley, J., Khanom, H. (2002) *Forced Marriage in the Bangladeshi Community*. London: Queen Mary, University of London.

Farmer, E., Parker, R. (1991) *Trials and Tribulations: Returning Children from Local Authority Care to Their Families*. London: HMSO.

Farrell, C. (1978) *My Mother Said: The Way Young People Learned About Sex and Birth Control*. London: Routledge.

Farrington, D. (2006) *Preventing Crime: What Works for Children, Offenders, Victims and Places*. New York: Springer.

Fergusson, D., Horwood, J., Lynskey, M. (1994) 'The childhoods of multiple problem adolescents: a 15 year longitudinal study'. *Journal of Child Psychology and Psychiatry*, 35:1123–1140.

Field, F. and White, P. (2007) *Welfare Isn t Working: The New Deal for Young People*. London: Reform.

Finney, A. (2006) *Domestic Violence, Sexual Assault and Stalking: Findings from the 2004/05 British Crime Survey Home Office Report 12/06*. Home Office. Available from: www.homeoffice.gov.uk/rds (accessed 23 March 2009).

Fonagy, P. (with Target, M., Cottrell, D., Phillips, J., Kurtz, Z.) (2002) *What Works for Whom? A Critical Review of Treatments for Children and Adolescents*. New York: Guilford.

Foshee, V.A., Linder, F., Macdougall, J.E., Bangdiwala, S. (2001) 'Gender differences in the longitudinal predictors of adolescent dating violence'. *Preventative Medicine*, 32:128–141.

Furnham, A., Husain, K. (1999) 'The role of conflict with parents in disordered eating among British Asian females'. *Social Psychiatry and Psychiatric Epidemiology*, 34 (9):498–505.

Gill, T. (2007) *No Fear: Growing Up in a Risk Averse Society*. London: Calouste Gaulbenkin Foundation.

Gillies, V. (2000) 'Young people and family life: Analysing and comparing disciplinary discourses'. *Journal of Youth Studies*, 3(2):211–228.

Gilligan, R. (1999) 'Enhancing the resilience of children in public care by mentoring their talent and interests'. *Child and Family Social Work*, 4(3):187–196.

Gilroy, P. (1987) *There Ain't No Black in the Union Jack*. London: Hutchinson.

Goldson, B., Lavalette, M., Mckechnie, J. (eds) (2002) *Children, Welfare and the State*. London: Sage.

Gorham, D. (1978) 'The "Maiden tribute of modern Babylon" re-examined: Child prostitution and the idea of childhood in late Victorian England'. *Victorian Studies*, 21 (3):353–379.

Greater London Authority (2007) *Demography Update October 2007*. Data Management and Analysis Group. London: Greater London Authority.

Green, J. (1992) *It's No Game*. Leicester: National Youth Agency.

Green, J., Mulroy, S., O'Neill, M. (1997) 'Young people and prostitution from a youth service perspective', in Barrett, D. (ed.). *Op Cit*.

Greenson, R.R. (1967) *The Technique and Practice of Psychoanalysis*. London: Hogarth Press.

Hackett, S. (2004) *What Works with Children and Young People with Harmful Sexual Behaviours*. Barkingside: Barnardo's.

Halpern, C., Young, M., Waller, M., Martin, S., Kupper, L. (2004) 'Prevalence of partner violence in same-sex romantic and sexual relationships in a national sample of adolescents'. *Journal of Adolescent Health*, 35:124–131.

Hammersley, M., Atkinson, P. (1993) *Ethnography: Principles in Practice*. 2nd Edition. London: Routledge.

Harbin, H.T., Madden, D.J. (1997) 'Battered parents: A new syndrome. *American Journal of Psychiatry*, 136(10):1288–1291.

Harker, L. (2006) *Chance of a Lifetime: The Impact of Bad Housing on Children's Lives*. London: Shelter.

Harper, Z., Scott, S. (2005) *Meeting the Needs of Sexually Exploited Young People in London*. Barkingside: Barnardo's.

Harrikson, S., Rickert, V., Wiemann, C. (2002) 'Prevalence and patterns of intimate partner violence among adolescent mothers during the postpartum period'. *Archives of Pediatrics and Adolescent Medicine*, 157(4):325–330.

Harris, J., Robinson, B. (2007) *Tipping the Iceberg: A Pan Sussex Study of Young People at Risk of Sexual Exploitation and Trafficking*. London: Barnardos.

Hart, R. (1997) *Children's Participation: The Theory and Practice of Involving Young Citizens in Community Development and Environmental Care*. New York: UNICEF.

Hayden, C. (2007) *Children in Trouble: The Role of Families, Schools and Communities*. Basingstoke: Palgrave.

Health Protection Agency, Scottish Centre for Infection and Environmental Health and Institute of Child Health (2004) *AIDS/HIV Quarterly Surveillance Tables, Cumulative Data to End June 2004*.

Hester, M., Westermarland, N. (2004) *Tackling Street Prostitution: Towards an Holistic Approach*. Home Office Research Study 279. London: Home Office.

Hester, M., Westmarland, N. (2005) *Tackling Domestic Violence: Effective Interventions and Approaches*. Home Office Research Study 290. London: Home Office Research, Development and Statistics Directorate.

Hester, M., Westmarland, N. (2006) *Service Provision for Perpetrators of Domestic Violence*. Bristol: University of Bristol.

Hill, M. (1990) 'The manifest and latent lessons of *child abuse enquiries'. British Journal of Social Work*, XX:197–213.

Hinsliff, G. (2004) *Men Who Fund Sex Traffic will be Criminalised. The Observer*, 21 November, 7.

Hobbs, D. (2001) 'Ethnography and the study of deviance', in Atkinson, P., Coffey, A., Delamont, S., Lofland, J., Lofland, L. (eds) *Handbook of Ethnography*. London: Sage Publications.

Hoggart, L. (2006) 'Risk: Young women and sexual decision-making [55 paragraphs]. *Forum Qualitative Sozialforschung/Forum: Qualitative Social Research* [online journal]. 7(1):Art. 28. Available from: www.qualitative-research.net/fqs-texte/1-06/06-1-28-e.htm (accessed 23 March 2009).

Holloway, W., Jefferson, T. (2000) *Doing Qualitative Research Differently: Free Association, Narrative and the Interview Method*. London: Sage.

HMSO (2007) *Cross Government Action Plan on Sexual Violence and Abuse*. London: HMSO.

HM Treasury (2008) *Ending Child Poverty: Every Bodies Business*. London: HM Treasury.

Home Office (2000) *Achieving Best Evidence in Criminal Proceedings: Guidance For Vulnerable or Intimidated Witnesses Including Children*. London: Home Office.

—— (2003) *Sexual Offences Act 2003, Chapter 42*. London: the Stationary Office. Available from: www.opsi.gov.uk/acts/acts2003 (accessed 23 March 2009).

—— (2004) *Paying the Price*. London: The Stationary Office.

—— (2005) *Domestic Violence: A National Report*. Home Office HMSO. Available from: www.crimereduction.homeoffice.gov.uk (accessed 23 March 2009).

—— (2006a) *Respect Action Plan*. Available from: www.homeoffice.gov.uk/documents/respect-action-plan (accessed 23 March 2009).

—— (2006b) *A Coordinated Prostitution Strategy*. London: HM Government.

—— (2006c) *Specialist Domestic Violence Court Programme Resource Manual*. London: HO HMSO.

—— (2007a) *A Guide to Anti-social Behaviour and Acceptable Behaviour*. Available from: www.crimereduction.homeoffice.gove.uk/asbos/asbos9.htm (accessed 23 March 2009).

—— (2007b) *Cutting Crime: A New Partnership Approach 2008 – 2011*. London: Home Office. Available from: www.crimereduction.homeoffice.gov.uk/crimereduction015. htm (accessed 21 April 2009).

—— (2008a) *Saving Lives: Reducing Harm. Protecting the Public. An Action Plan for Tackling Violence 2008-2011*. London: Home Office. Available from: www.crimer-eduction.homeoffice.gov.uk/domesticviolence/domesticviolence069a.pdf (accessed 21 April 2009).

—— (2008b) *Drugs: Protecting Families and Communities. The 2008 Drug Strategy*. London: Home Office, HMSO.

Home Office and the Scottish Government (2007) *UK Action Plan in Tackling Human Trafficking*. London: HO/HMSO.

—— (2008) *Update to the UK Human Trafficking Action Plan July 2008*. London: Home Office. Available from: www.crimereduction.homeoffice.gov.uk/humantrafficking004. pdf (accessed 21 April 2009).

Howard, S., Dryden, J., Johnson, B. (1999) 'Childhood resilience: Review and critique of literature'. *Oxford Review of Education*, 25(3):307–323.

Howe, D. (1998) 'Relationship-based thinking and practice in social work'. *Journal of Social Work Practice*, 1(12):45–56.

—— (2005) *Child Abuse and Neglect. Attachment, Development and Intervention*. Basingstoke: Palgrave.

Hudson, A. (1988) 'Boys will be boys: Masculinism and the juvenile justice system'. *Critical Social Policy*, 21:30–48.

Hunter, G., May, T. (2004) *Solutions and Strategies: Drug Problems and Street Sex Markets- Guidance for Partnerships and Providers*. London: Home Office.

Hynes, P. (2009) 'Contemporary compulsory dispersal and the absence of space for the restoration of trust'. *Journal of Refugee Studies*, 22(1): 97–121.

Irwin, C.E. Jr., Millstein, S.G. (1986) 'Biopsychosocial correlates of risk-taking beha-viours during adolescence'. *Journal of Adolescent Health Care*, 7:82–96.

Israel, M., Hay, I. (2006) *Research Ethics in the Social Sciences*. London: Sage Publications.

Itzin, C. (2008) *Tackling the Root Causes of Mental Illness in Domestic and Sexual Violence and Abuse. A Compendium of Guidelines and Information on Therapeutic and Preventative Interventions with Victims, Survivors and Abusers, Children, Ado-lescents and Adults*. London: Department of Health.

Izzidien, S. (2008) *I Can't Tell People What is Happening at Home. Domestic Abuse within South Asian Communities: The Specific Needs of Women, Children and Young People*. London: NSPCC Inform.

Jago, S., Pearce, J. (2008) *Gathering Evidence of the Sexual Exploitation of Children and Young People: A Scoping Exercise*. Luton: University of Bedfordshire.

Jeffs, T., Smith, M. (2002) 'Individualisation and youth work'. *Youth and Policy*, 76:39–66.

Jesson, J. (1993) 'Understanding adolescent female prostitution: A literature review'. *British Journal of Social Work*, 23:517–530.

Jessor, R., Jessor, S. (1977) *Problem Behaviour and Psychosocial Development: A Long-itudinal Study of Youth*. New York: Academic Press.

Jessor, R., Turbin, M.S., Costa, F.M., QiDong, H.Z., Wang, C. (2003) 'Adolescent problem behaviour in China and the United States: A cross national study of psycho-social protective factors'. *Journal of Research on Adolescence*, 13:329–360.

Jones, H., MacGregor, S. (1998) *Social Issues and Party Politics*. London: Routledge.

Joseph Rowntree Foundation (2006) *What Will It Take to End Child Poverty?* www.jrf. org.uk/child poverty (accessed 21 April 2009).

Kaestle, C., Halpern, C. (2005) 'Sexual intercourse precedes partner violence in adolescent romantic relationships'. *Journal of Adolescent Health*, 36:386–392.

Kaestle, C.E., Halpern, C.T., Hallfors, D., Waller, M., Iritani, B. (2004) *Early Pubertal Timing, Age of Romantic Partners, and HIV Risk Behaviors*. Poster presented at Society for Research on Adolescence (SRA) Biennial Meeting, Baltimore, Maryland.

Kelly, L., Regan, L., Burton, S. (2000b) 'Sexual exploitation: A new discovery or one part of the continuum of sexual abuse in childhood?', in Itzin, C. (ed.) *Home Truths About Child Sexual Abuse: Influencing Policy and Practice a Reader*. London: Routledge.

King, R., Skeldon, R., Vullentari, J. (2008) *Internal and International Migration: Bridging the Theoretical Divide*. Brighton: Sussex Centre for Migration, University of Sussex.

Kinnell, H. (2008) *Violence and Sex Work in Britain*. Devon: Willan Publishing.

Kirby, P. (1995) *A Word from the Street: Young People Who Leave Care and Become Homeless*. London: Centre Point and Community Care/Reed Publishing.

Kohli, R., Mather, R. (2003) 'Promoting psychosocial well being in unaccompanied asylum seeking young people in the United Kingdom'. *Child and Family Social Work*, 8:201–212.

Kumagai, F. (1981) 'Filial violence: A peculiar parent-child relationship in the Japanese family today'. *Journal of Comparative Family Studies*, XII(3):337–350.

Kyle, A. (2008) *Sexual Exploitation of Boys Sask.'s Dark Secret: Report. Canwest News Service*, Monday, 1 December 2008.

Lane, P., Tribe, R. (2006) 'Unequal care: An introduction to understanding UK policy and the impact on asylum-seeking children'. *International Journal of Migration, Health and Social Care*, 2(2):7–14.

Langan, M., Lee, P. (1989) *Radical Social Work Today*. London: Unwin Hyman.

Leboch, E., King, S. (2006) 'Child sexual exploitation: A partnership response and model intervention'. *Child Abuse Review*, 15(5):362–372.

Lee, M., O'Brien, R. (1995) *The Game's Up: Redefining Child Prostitution*. London: The Children's Society.

Lee, R.M. (1993) *Doing Research on Sensitive Topics*. London: Sage Publications.

Lees, S. (2002) 'Gender, ethnicity and vulnerability in young women in local authority care'. *British Journal of Social Work*, 32:907–922.

Lee-treweek, G., Linkogle, S. (2000) *Danger in the Field: Risk and Ethics in Social Research*. London: Routledge.

Lester, H., Glasby, J. (2006) *Mental Health Policy and Practice*. London: Palgrave Macmillan.

Lewis, E., Martinez, A. (2006) *Addressing Healthy Relationships and Sexual Exploitation within PSHE in Schools*. Sex Education Forum Fact Sheet 37. London: National Children's Bureau.

Lillywhite, R., Skidmore, P. (2006) 'Boys are not sexually exploited? A challenge to practitioners'. *Child Abuse Review*, 15:351–361.

London Assembly (2005) *Street Prostitution in London*. London. Available from: www/london.gov.uk/assembly/reports/pubserv.jsp (accessed 23 March 2009).

Luthar, S.S. (ed.) (2003) *Resilience and Vulnerability: Adaptation in the Context of Childhood Adversities*. Cambridge: Cambridge University Press.

Luxmoore, N. (2008) *Feeling like Crap: Young People and the Meaning of Self Esteem*. London: Jessica Kingsley Publishers.

Macfarlane, A., McPherson, A. (1999) *Teenagers, the Agony, the Ecstasy, the Answers*. London: Warner Books.

Macfie, J., Cicchetti, D., Toth, S. (2001) 'The development of dissociation in maltreated pre-school children'. *Development and Psychopathology*, 13:233–254.

Masud Ali, A.K.M., Sarkar, R. in collaboration with INCIDIN Bangladesh (2006) *The Boys and the Bullies: A Situational Analysis Report on Prostitution of Boys in Bangladesh*. ECPAT International and INCIDIN Bangladesh. Available from: www.humantrafficking.org (accessed 23 March 2009).

Mauthner, M., Birch, J., Jessop, J., Miller, T. (eds) (2002) *Ethics in Qualitative Research*. pp. 107–122. London: Sage Publications.

May, T., Edmunds, M. and Hough, M. (1999) *Street Business: The Links Between Sex Markets and Drug Markets*. London: Police Research Series, Paper 134.

McKeganey, N., Barnard, M. (1996) *Sex Work on the Streets*. Milton Keynes: Open University Press.

McMullen, R.J. (1987) 'Youth prostitution; a balance of power'. *Journal of Adolescence*, 10(1):35–43.

McMullen, R.J. (1988) 'Boys involved in prostitution'. *Youth and Policy*, 23:35–41.

McRobbie, A. (1991) *Feminism and Youth Culture: from Jackie to Just Seventeen*. Boston: Allan and Unwin.

Meetoo, V., Mirza, H. (2007) 'Lives at risk: Multiculturalism, young women and "honour" killings', in Thom, B., Sales, R., Pearce, J. (eds), *Growing Up with Risk*. London: Policy Press.

Melrose, M. (2002) 'Labour pains: Some considerations of the difficulties in researching juvenile prostitution'. *International Journal of Social Research Theory, Methodology and Practice*, 5(4):333–352.

Melrose, M. (ed.) with Barrett, D. (2004) *Anchors in Floating Lives; Interventions with Young People Sexually Abused Through Prostitution*. Lyme Regis: Russell House Publishing.

Melrose, M., Barett, D., Brodie, I. (1999) *One Way Street? Retrospectives on Childhood Prostitution*. London: The Children's Society and University of Luton.

Mirza, H. (1992) *Young, Female and Black*. London: Routledge.

—— (2007) 'Multiculturalism and the gender trap: Young ethnicised women and domestic violence in schools'. *Education Review*, 20(2):46–56.

Mitchell, F. (2004) *Living in Limbo: Survey of Homeless Households Living in Temporary Accommodation*. London: Shelter.

Mooney, J. (2000) *Gender, Violence and the Social Order*. London: Palgrave Macmillan.

Moore, S.M., Rosenthal, D.A. (1992) 'Adolescent sexuality, social contexts: safe sex implications'. *Journal of Adolescence*, 15:415–435.

—— (2006) *Sexuality in Adolescence, Current Trends*. London: Routledge.

Morris, J., Paulson, Robert, H., Coombs, I., Landsverk, J. (1990) 'Youth who physically assault their parents'. *Journal of Family Violence*, 5(2):121–133.

Munro, C. (2004) *Scratching the Surface … What We Know About the Abuse and Sexual Exploitation of Young People by Adults Targeting Residential and Supported Accommodation Units*. Unpublished paper, Barnardo's Street Team, Glasgow.

Murray, C. (2005) 'Children and young people's participation and non participation in research'. *Adoption and Fostering*, 29(1):57–66.

Narey, M. (2006) *Reducing the Risk: Barnardo's Support For Sexually Exploited Young People*. London: Barnardos.

National Youth Agency (2008) *Reconnecting Detached Youth Work: Guidelines and Standards for Excellence*. Leicester: The Federation for Detached Youth Work, NYA.

Newman, T. (2002) *Promoting Resilience in Children and Young People During Periods of Transition*. Edinburgh: Scottish Executive. Available from: www.scotland.gov.uk/library5/education/ic78-00.asp (accessed 23 March 2009).

—— (2004) *What Works in Building Resilience*. Ilford: Barnados.

Newman, T., Blackburn, S. (2002) *Transitions in the Lives of Children and Young People: Resilience Factors*. Edinburgh: The Scottish Government.

Newburn, T., Shiner, M. (2005) *Dealing with Disaffection: Young People, Mentoring and Social Inclusion*. Devon: Willan Publishing.

NHS Health Scotland (2005) *Young People's Attitudes Towards Gendered Violence-August 2005*. Edinburgh: NHS Health Scotland.

Nottingham (2005) *Nottinghamshire's Children's Fund Domestic Violence: Children's Outreach Services: Evaluation Summary*. Nottingham Local Authority.

NSPCC (2004) *Street Matters Project*. London: NSPCC.

NWG (2008) *2007-2008 Annual Report*. Available from: www.nationalworkinggroup.co.uk (accessed 23 March 2009).

O'Brien, L. (1995) *The Games Up*. London: The Children's Society.

O'Connell, R. (2003) *A Typology of Child Cybersexploitation and Online Grooming Practices*. Preston: University of Central Lancashire.

O'Connell-Davidson, J. (2002) *Prostitution, Power and Freedom*. Cambridge: Polity Press.

—— (2005a) *Men, Middlemen and Migrants*. Cambridge: Polity.

—— (2005b) *Children in the Global Sex Trade*. Cambridge, Malden: Polity Press.

Okin, S.M. (1999) *Is Multiculturalism Bad for Women*. Available from: www.bostonreview.net (accessed 23 March 2009).

Omer, H. (2004) *Nonviolent Resistance a New Approach to Violent and Self Destructive Children*. Cambridge: University Press.

Pain, R., Francis, P., Fuller, I., O'Brien, K., Williams, S. (2002) 'Hard-to-reach young people and community safety: A model for participatory research and consultation'. *Police Research Series*, Paper 152.

Palmer, T. (2001) *No Son of Mine! Children Abused Through Prostitution*. Barkingside: Barnardo's.

Palmer, T., Stacey, L. (2004) *Just One Click*. Barkingside: Barnardo's.

Paterson, R., Luntz, H., Perlesz, A., Cotton, S. (2002) 'Adolescent violence towards parents maintaining family connections when the going gets tough'. *Australian and New Zealand Journal of Family Therapy*, 23(2):90–100.

Peacock, D., Rothman, E. (2001) *Working with Young Men Who Batter: Current Strategies and New Directions*. Harrisburg, Pennsylvania: VAWnet, a project of the National Resource Center on Domestic Violence/Pennsylvania Coalition Against Domestic Violence. Available from: www.vawnet.org (accessed 23 March 2009).

Pearce, J. and Street Reach (2009) *Our Stories: Out of the Box: Young People's Accounts of Sexual Exploitation*. Luton: Bedfordshire University.

Pearce, J. (2009 forthcoming) *Young People, Poverty, Social Exclusion and Sexual Exploitation*. In Phoenix, J. (ed.) *Regulating Sex for Sale: Prostitution, Policy Reform and the UK*. Bristol: Policy Press.

Pearce, J., Hynes, P., Bovarnick, S. (2009) *Practitioners Responses to Trafficked Children and Young People*. London: NSPCC.

Pearce, J., with Williams, M., Galvin, C. (2002). *It's Someone Taking a Part of You; A Study of Young Women and Sexual Exploitation*. London: National Children's Bureau.

Pearce, J.J. (1999) 'Selling sex, doing drugs and keeping safe', in Marlow, A., Pearson, G. (eds) *Young People, Drugs and Community Safety.* pp. 118–127. Lyme Regis: Russell House Publishing.

—— (2000) 'Young people and sexual exploitation: A European issue'. *Social Work in Europe*, 7:24–30.

—— (2006a) 'Who needs to be involved in safeguarding sexually exploited young people?' *Child Abuse Review*, 5(5):326–341.

—— (2006b) 'Finding the "I" in sexual exploitation: hearing the voices of sexually exploited young people in policy and practice', in Campbell, R. O'Neill, M. (eds) *Sex Work Now.* pp. 190–212. Cullompton, Devon: Willan Press.

—— (2007a) 'Risk and resilience: A focus on sexually exploited young people', in Thom, B., Sales, R., Pearce, J. (eds) *Growing Up with Risk.* London: Policy Press.

—— (2007b) 'Sex and risk', in Coleman, J., Hagell, A. (eds) *Adolescence, Risk and Resilience: Against the Odds.* pp. 63–89. London: John Wiley.

Pearson, G. (1983) *Hooligan: A History of Respectable Fears.* London: Macmillan.

—— (1993) 'Forward', in Hobbs, D., May, T. (eds) *Interpreting the Field: Accounts of Ethnography.* Oxford: Clarendon Press.

Peek, C, Fisher, J. et al (1985) 'Teenage violence towards parents. A neglected dimension of family violence'. *Journal of Marriage and the Family*, 47:1051–1058.

Phoenix, J. (1994) *Making Sense of Prostitution.* Hampshire: Macmillan.

—— (2002) 'In the name of protection: Youth prostitution policy reforms in England and Wales'. *Critical Social Policy*, 22(2):353–375.

—— (2004) 'Regulating sex: Young people, prostitution and policy reform', in Brookes-Gordon, B., Gelsthorpe, L., Johnson, M., Bainham, A. (eds) *Sexuality Repositioned*, Oxford: Hart Publishing.

—— (ed.) (2009) *Regulating Sex for Sale: Prostitution, Policy Reform and the UK.* Bristol: Policy Press.

Phoenix, J., Oerton, S. (2005) *Illicit and Illegal: Sex, Regulation and Social Control.* Devon: Willan Publishing.

Picklington, J., Lothian, F. (2007) *Friend or Foe.* Sheffield: Sheffield Taking Stock.

Pitts, J. (1997) 'Causes of prostitution, new forms of practice and political responses', in Barrett D. (ed.) *Child Prostitution in Britain: Dilemmas and Practical Responses.* pp. 139–158. London: The Children's Society.

—— (2008) *Reluctant Gangers.* Cullompton, Devon: Willan Press.

Poudel, P., Carryer, J. (2000) 'Girl-trafficking, HIV/AIDS and the position of women in Napal'. *Gender and Development*, 8(2):74–79.

Rafferty, Y. (2007) 'Children for sale: Child trafficking in Southeast Asia'. *Child Abuse Review*, 16:401–422.

Rathbone (2008) *Engaging Youth Enquiry 2007-2008. New Approaches to Engaging Youth: Understanding the Problems and Implementing the Solutions. Rathbone/Nuffield 14-19 Review.* Manchester: Rathbone.

Rice, B. (2006) *Against the Odds.* London: Shelter.

Riess, D., Richards, J.E., Radke-Yarrow, M., Scharff, D. (1993) *Children and Violence.* London: Guildford Press.

Riger, S, Wasco, S., Schewe, P. (2002) *Evaluating Services for Survivors of Domestic Violence and Sexual Assault.* London: Sage.

Ronker, A., Oravala, S., Pulkinner, L. (2002) 'I met this wife of mine, and things got on a better track'. Turning points in risk development. *Journal of Adolescence*, 25:47–64.

Rotherham Local Safeguarding Children Board (2008) 'Annual report on protection of young people in Rotherham from sexual exploitation'. Rotherham.

Ruggiero, V., Montagna, N. (2008) *Social Movements: A Reader*. London: Routledge.

Rutherford, A. (1986) *Growing Out of Crime: Society and Young People in Trouble*. Middlesex: Penguin Books.

Rutter, M. (1985) 'Resilience in the face of adversity: Protective factors and resilience to psychiatric disorders'. *British Journal of Psychiatry*, 147:589–611.

Rutter, M., Taylor, E. (2002) *Child and Adolescent Psychiatry*. Blackwell Publishing.

Sanders, T. (2005) *Sex Work: A Risky Business*. Devon: William Press.

Sanders, T.L.M. (2008) *Paying for Pleasure: Men Who Buy Sex*. Cullompton, Devon: Willan.

Save the Children, Sweden (Radda Barnen) (2005) *The Client Goes Unnoticed*. Stockholm: Save The Children Sweden. Available from: www.rb.se (accessed 23 March 2009).

Savin-Williams, R.C., Diamond, L. (2001) 'Sexual identity trajectories among sexual minority youths: Gender comparisons'. *Archives of Sexual Behaviour*, 29:419–440.

Schutt, N. (2006) *Domestic Violence in Adolescent Relationships*. London: Safer Southwark Partnerships.

Scott, S., Harper, Z. (2006) 'Meeting the needs of sexually exploited Young people: the challenge of conducting policy relevant research'. *Child Abuse Review*, 15:313–325.

Scott, S., Skidmore, P. (2006) *Reducing the Risk: Barnardo's Support For Sexually Exploited Young People*. London: Barnardo's.

Self, H. (2003) *Prostitution, Women and the Misuse of the Law: The Fallen Daughters of Eve*. London: Franck Cass.

Sexually Exploited Children Outreach Service (SECOS) (2008) *What We Do*. Available from: www.barnardos.org.uk/secos (accessed 23 March 2009).

Sharland, E. (2005) 'Young people, risk taking and risk making: Some thoughts for social work'. *British Journal of Social Work*, 36: 247–265.

Sharpe, S. (1977) *Just Like a Girl: How Girls Learn to Become Women*. Harmonsworth: Penguin.

Sheehan, M. (1997) 'Adolescent violence-strategies, outcomes and dilemmas in working with young people and their families'. *Australian and New Zealand Journal of Family Therapy*, 18(2):80–91.

Sheffield (2006) *Sheffield Safeguarding Children Board: Sexual Exploitation Service 2005-2006*. Sheffield: Sheffield Safeguarding Children Board.

Sheffield (2008) *Sexual Exploitation Service*. Available from: www.safeguardingsheffield children.org.uk/welcome/safeguarding-children-board/sexual-exploitation (accessed 21 April 2009).

Sheffield Safeguarding Children Board (2007) *Sexual Exploitation Service 2006-2007*. Sheffield: Sheffield Safeguarding Children Board.

Shelter (2008) *Supporting Children and Families*. Available from: www.shelter.org.uk (accessed 23 March 2009).

Shildrick, T., MacDonald, R. (2008) 'Understanding youth exclusion: critical moments, social networks and social capital'. *Youth and Policy*, 99:43–55.

Silverman, D. (2006) *Interpreting Qualitative Data*. 3rd Edition. London: Sage.

Singh Ghuman, P. (2003) *Double Loyalties: South Asian Adolescents in the West*. Cardiff: University of Wales Press.

Skelton, T., Valentine, G. (1998) *Cool Places: Geographies of Youth Cultures*. London: Routledge.

Skidmore, P. (1999) *Nottingham Child Prostitution Pilot Study; Report to the Policing and Reducing Crime Unit, Home Office*. London and Nottingham: London Guildhall University and Nottingham Trent University.

Skidmore, P., Lillywhite, R. (2006) 'Boys are not sexually exploited? A challenge to practitioners'. *Child Abuse Review*, 15(5):351–361.

Skinner, T., Hester, M., Malos, E. (eds) (2005) *Researching Gender Violence: Feminist Methodology in Action*. Devon: Willan Publishing.

Social Exclusion Unit (2005) *Transitions: A Social Exclusion Unit Interim Report on Young Adults*. London: Office of the Deputy Prime Minister Social Exclusion Unit.

Somerset, C. (2001) *What the Professionals Know: The Trafficking of Children into, and Through the UK for Sexual Purposes*. London: ECPAT UK.

—— (2004) *Cause for Concern: London Social Services and Child Trafficking*. London: End Child Prostitution and Trafficking, UK.

Sprott, J.B., Doob, A.N. (2000) 'Bad, sad and rejected: The lives of aggressive children'. *Canadian Journal of Criminology*, 42(2):123–133.

Stanko, E. (1998) *Taking Stock: What Do We Know About Violence? ESRC Violence Programme*. London: Brunel University.

Street Reach (2007) *Street Reach Annual Report 2006 – 2007*. Available from: www. streetreach.org.uk (accessed 23 March 2009).

Swan Housing Group (2007) *Look Again: Annual Report 2006/7*. Available from: www. swan.org.uk (accessed 23 March 2009).

Swann, S. (2008) 'Using the Sexual Offences Act 2003 to protect sexually exploited children and young people'. *Conference presentation at Safe and Sound Derby and National Working Group for Sexually Exploited Children and Young People (NWG)*. Derby.

Swann, S., Balding, V. (2002) *Safeguarding Children Involved in Prostitution: Guidance Review*. Available from: www.doh.uk/acpc/safeguardingchildrenreview.pdf (accessed 23 March 2009).

Swann, S., McNosh, D., Edwards, S. (1998) *Whose Daughter Next? Children Abused Through Prostitution*. London: Barnardos.

Taylor-Browne, J. (2002) *More Than One Chance: Young People Involved in Prostitution Speak Out*. London: ECPAT.

The Children's Society (2008) *Stepping Up: The Future of Runaways Services*. London: The Children's Society.

The National Working Group for Sexually Exploited Children and Young People (2008) *Annual Report*. Available from: www.nationalworkinggroup.co.uk (accessed 21 April 2009).

Trickett, P. (1997) 'Sexual and physical abuse and the development of social competence', in Luthar, S., Burack, J., Cicchetti, D., Weisze, I.J. (eds) *Developmental Psychopathology: Perspectives on Adjustment, Risk and Disorder*. pp. 67–92. New York: Cambridge University Press.

Trickett, P., Putman, F. (1998) 'Developmental consequences of child sexual abuse', in Trickett, P., Schellenbach, C. (eds) *Violence Against Children in the Family and the Community*. pp. 39–56. Washington DC: American Psychological Association.

Triesman, A.E., Whittaker, J.K., Brendtro, L.K. (1969) *The Other 23 Hours: Childcare Work with Emotionally Disturbed Children in a Therapeutic Milieu*. New York: Hawthorne.

Troiden, R.R. (1989) 'The formation of homosexual identities', in Herdt, G. (ed.) *Gay and Lesbian Youth*, New York: Hanworth Press.

UKNSWP (2007) *Directory of Services 2007/8*. Manchester: UKNSWP. Available from: www.uknswp.co.uk (accessed 21 April 2009).
—— (2008) UK Network of Sex Work Projects. Available from: www.uknswp.org (accessed 21 April 2009).
UNICEF (with the Office of the High Commissioner for Human Rights (OHCHR) and the OSCE Office for Democratic Institutions and Human Rights (ODIHR) (2005) *Trafficking in Human Beings in South Eastern Europe*. Geneva: UNICEF.
UNICEF and ECPAT (2007) *Rights Here, Rights now*. London: ECPAT UK.
United Kingdom Border Agency (UKBA) (2007) *Code of Practice For Keeping Children Safe from Harm: Section 21 of the UK Borders Act 2007 UK*. London: BA.
United National Children Fund (UNICEF) and Terre des Hommes (2006) *Action to Prevent Child Trafficking in South Eastern Europe: A Preliminary Assessment*. Geneva: UNICEF.
United Nations (1989) *Convention on the Rights of the Child*. Geneva: UN Office of the High Commissioner for Human Rights.
—— (2003) *The Palermo Protocol: to Prevent, Suppress and Punish Trafficking in Persons, Especially Women and Children*. Geneva: UN.
US Department of State (2007) *Victims of Trafficking and Violence Protection Act of 2000: Trafficking in Persons report 2007*. Available from: www.state.gov/g/tip/rls/tiprpt/2007 (accessed 23 March 2009).
Utting, W. (1997) *People Like Us: The Report of the Review of the Safeguards for Children Living Away from Home*. London: The Stationary Office.
Valentine, G., Skelton, T., Butler, R. (2002) 'The vulnerability and marginalisation of lesbian and gay youth'. *Youth and Policy*, 75:4–29.
Varma, V. (1997) *Violence in Children & Adolescents*. London: Jessica Kingsley.
Walby, Allen (2004) *Domestic Violence, Sexual Assault and Stalking: Findings from the British Crime Survey*. Home Office Research, Development and Statistics Directorate.
Walkowitz, J. (1992) *City of Dreadful Delight: Narratives of Sexual Danger in Late Victorian London*. London: Virago Press.
Ward, A. (2003) 'Using everyday life: Opportunity led work', in Ward, A., Kasinski, K., Pooley, J., Worthington, A. (eds) *Therapeutic Communities For Children and Young People*. pp. 119–132. London: Jessica Kingsley.
Ward, A., Kasinski, K., Pooley, J., Worthington, A. (eds) (2003) *Therapeutic Communities for Children and Young People*. London: Jessica Kingsley.
Ward, J. (2008) 'Researching drug sellers: An "experiential" account from "the field"'. *Sociological Research Online*, 13(1). Available from: www.socresonline.org.uk/13/1/14.html (accessed 27 April 2009).
Ward, J., Bayley, M. (2007) 'Young people's perceptions of risk', in Thom, B., Sales, R., Pearce, J. (eds) *Growing Up with Risk*, pp. 37–57. Bristol: Policy Press.
Ward, J., Henderson, Z. (2003) 'Some practical and ethical issues encountered while conducting tracking research with young people leaving the "care" system'. *International Journal Social Research Methodology*, 6(3):255–259.
Ward, J., Patel, N. (2006) 'Broadening the discussion on "sexual exploitation": Ethnicity, sexual exploitation and young people', in Lowe, K. and Pearce, J. (eds) *Child Abuse Review: Themed Issue on Young People and Sexual Exploitation. Child Abuse Review*, 15(5):341–351.
Weinstock, A. (2007) *Targeted Youth Support Guide and the Fit with Integrated Youth Support Services*. DCSF. Available from: www.everychildmatters.gov.uk (accessed 27 April 2009).

Wellings, K., Nanchahal, K., Macdowall,W., McNanus, S., Erens, B., Mercer, C.H., Johnson, A.M., Copas, A.J., Korovessis, C., Fenton, K. (2001) 'Sexual behaviour in Britain: Early heterosexual experience'. *The Lancet*, 358:1843–1850.

West, D.J., with de Villiers, B. (1992) *Male Prostitution*. London: Duckworth.

Wheeler, R. (2006) 'Gillick or Fraser? A plea for consistency over competence in children'. *British Medical Journal*, 332(7545):807.

Whowell, M. and Gaffney J. (2009 forthcoming) 'Male sex work in the UK: Forms, practice and policy implications', in Phoenix, J. (ed.) *Regulating Sex for Sale: Prostitution, Policy Reform and the UK*. Bristol: Policy Press.

Wight, D., Henderson, M., Raab, G., Abraham, C., Buston, K., Scott, S., Hart, G. (2000) 'Extent of regretted sexual intercourse among young teenagers in Scotland'. *British Medical Journal*, 320:1243–1244.

Williamson, E., Goodenough, T. (2005) 'Conducting research with children: The limits of confidentiality and child protection protocols'. *Children and Society*, 19:397–409.

Willis, P. (1977) *Learning to Labour: How Working Class Kids Get Working Class Jobs*. Farnborough: Saxon House.

Wilson, P. (2003) 'Consultation and supervision', in Ward, A., Kasinski, K., Pooley, J., Worthington, A. (eds) *Therapeutic Communities For Children and Young People*. London: Jessica Kingsley.

Windfuhr, K., While, D., Hunt, I., Turnbull, P., Lowe, R., Burns, J., Swinson, N., Shaw, J., Appleby, L., Kapur, N. and the National Confidential Inquiry into Suicide and Homicide by People with Mental Illness. (2008) 'Suicide in juveniles and adolescents in the United Kingdom'. *Journal of Child Psychology and Psychiatry*, 49(11):1157–1167.

Women's Aid (2006) *Why Doesn't She Leave*. Available from: www.womensaid.org.uk/domestic-violence-articles.asp?section = 0001 (accessed 23 March 2009).

Yates, S., Payne, M. (2007) '"Minding the gap" between policy visions and service implementation: Lessons from Connexions'. *Youth and Policy Journal*, 95:25–31.

Zimmerman, C., Hossain, M., Yun, K., Roche, B., Morison, L., Watts, C. (2006) *Stolen Smiles: A Summary Report on the Physical and Psychological Health Consequences of Women and Adolescents Trafficked in Europe*. London: London School of Hygiene and Tropical Medicine.

Index

Abduction Act (1984) 76
abusers *see* perpetrators
accommodation: bed and breakfast 37–38, 44, 72; inadequacy of for homeless 37–38; need for supported 36–37, 72; provision of through partnership between local authorities and housing providers 38
ACPO *see* Association of Chief Police Officers
Action Plan on Sexual Violence and Abuse 122
adolescence: as a developmental life stage 16, 46
adolescent intimate personal violence (AIPV) 68–69
adolescents in violent partnerships (AVP) 5–6; and domestic violence 64–81
adulthood: transition from child to 16, 31, 64, 70, 71, 72, 86, 115, 147
Africa: source region for trafficking 55
'Aim high for young people' initiative 25
AIPV (adolescent intimate personal violence) 68–69
alcohol use 34, 36, 142–43, 149; linking with early sexual activity 87–88
antisocial behaviour 89; of sexually exploited children 13, 14–15
antisocial behaviour orders 90
Area Child Protection Committees (ACPCs) 26, 27–28, 106 *see also* Local Safeguarding Children Boards
Asian young women 129–30
Association of Chief Police Officers (ACPO) 22–23, 125
Association for Moral and Social Hygiene (AMSH) 16
attachment(s): and Barnardos four 'A's 146; centrality to recovery of good 156;

challenges to developing and maintaining 142, 147–48; developing of good 92–93, 149–51; role of good 148–49; *see also* relationship-based interventions
attachment disorder 35
Awaken Project (Blackpool) 107, 127

Baby P case 31, 65, 108
Balding, V. 27, 106
Bangladeshis 97, 98, 129, 130
Barnardos 30, 79, 131, 139, 147; and ethical issues in research 111, 118; evaluation of their services 14, 37, 94, 97, 107, 127; four 'A's 146–47; 'Sexually Exploited Children Outreach Services' (SECOS) project 40; Streets and Lanes Project 21; triangles 27, 28; 'Whose Daughter Next' campaign 21–22; Young Men's Project 125, 127
Barrett, D. 38
bed and breakfast accommodation 37–38, 44, 72
black and minority ethnic (BME) young people 67, 77–78, 126–30, 138; and children's services support 127, 130; and domestic violence 77; impact of risk factors on 129–30; running away from home 129–30; service provision for sexually exploited 77, 128–29; and sexual exploitation 78, 127–28
Blackburn, S. 91
'blame' culture 15, 18
Borders Act (2007) (UK) 47
Booth, Bramwell 12
Border and Immigration Agency (BIA) (now UK Border Agency) 47
boys, sexually exploited *see* young men/ boys, sexually exploited

DATE DUE